# The Association Between School-Based Physical Activity, Including Physical Education, and Academic Performance

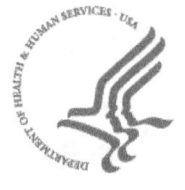

**U.S. Department of Health and Human Services**
Centers for Disease Control and Prevention
National Center for Chronic Disease Prevention and Health Promotion
Division of Adolescent and School Health
www.cdc.gov/HealthyYouth

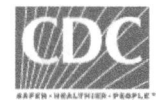

Revised Version — July 2010
(Replaces April 2010 Early Release)

***Acknowledgments:***
This publication was developed for the Centers for Disease Control and Prevention's (CDC) Division of Adolescent and School Health (DASH) under contract #200 2002-00800 with ETR Associates.

***Suggested Citation:***
Centers for Disease Control and Prevention. *The association between school based physical activity, including physical education, and academic performance.* Atlanta, GA: U.S. Department of Health and Human Services; 2010.

# TABLE OF CONTENTS

# EXECUTIVE SUMMARY

When children and adolescents participate in the recommended level of physical activity—at least 60 minutes daily—multiple health benefits accrue. Most youth, however, do not engage in recommended levels of physical activity. Schools provide a unique venue for youth to meet the activity recommendations, as they serve nearly 56 million youth. At the same time, schools face increasing challenges in allocating time for physical education and physical activity during the school day.

There is a growing body of research focused on the association between school-based physical activity, including physical education, and academic performance among school-aged youth. To better understand these connections, this review includes studies from a range of physical activity contexts, including school-based physical education, recess, classroom-based physical activity (outside of physical education and recess), and extracurricular physical activity. The purpose of this report is to synthesize the scientific literature that has examined the association between school-based physical activity, including physical education, and academic performance, including indicators of cognitive skills and attitudes, academic behaviors, and academic achievement.

## Methods

For this review, relevant research articles and reports were identified through a search of nine electronic databases, using both physical activity and academic-related search terms. The search yielded a total of 406 articles that were examined to determine their match with the inclusion criteria. Forty-three articles (reporting a total of 50 unique studies) met the inclusion criteria and were read, abstracted, and coded for this synthesis.

Coded data from the articles were used to categorize and organize studies first by their physical activity context (i.e., physical education, recess, classroom-based physical activity, and extracurricular physical activities), and then by type of academic performance outcome. Academic performance outcomes were grouped into three categories: 1) academic achievement (e.g.,

grades, test scores); 2) academic behavior (e.g., on-task behavior, attendance); and 3) cognitive skills and attitudes (e.g., attention/concentration, memory, mood). Findings of the 43 articles that explored the relationship between indicators of physical activity and academic performance were then summarized.

## Results

Across all 50 studies (reported in 43 articles), there were a total of 251 associations between physical activity and academic performance, representing measures of academic achievement, academic behavior, and cognitive skills and attitudes. Measures of cognitive skills and attitudes were used most frequently (112 of the 251 associations tested). Of all the associations examined, slightly more than half (50.5%) were positive, 48% were not significant, and only 1.5% were negative. Examination of the findings by each physical activity context provided insights regarding specific relationships.

### 1) *School-Based Physical Education Studies*

School-based physical education as a context category encompassed 14 studies (reported in 14 articles) that examined physical education courses or physical activity conducted in physical education class. Typically, these studies examined the impact of increasing the amount of time students spent in physical education class or manipulating the activities during physical education class. Overall, increased time in physical education appears to have a positive relationship or no relationship with academic achievement. Increased time in physical education does not appear to have a negative relationship with academic achievement. Eleven of the 14 studies found one or more positive associations between school-based physical education and indicators of academic performance; the remaining three studies found no significant associations.

### 2) *Recess Studies*

Eight recess studies (reported in six articles) explored the relationship between academic performance and recess during the school day in elementary schools. Six studies tested an intervention to examine how recess impacts indicators of academic performance;

the other two studies explored the relationships between recess and school adjustment or classroom behavior. Time spent in recess appears to have a positive relationship with, or no relationship with, children's attention, concentration, and/or on-task classroom behavior. All eight studies found one or more positive associations between recess and indicators of cognitive skills, attitudes, and academic behavior; none of the studies found negative associations.

### 3) Classroom Physical Activity Studies

Nine studies (reported in nine articles) explored physical activity that occurred in classrooms apart from physical education classes and recess. In general, these studies explored short physical activity breaks (5–20 minutes) or ways to introduce physical activity into learning activities that were either designed to promote learning through physical activity or provide students with a pure physical activity break. These studies examined how the introduction of brief physical activities in a classroom setting affected cognitive skills (aptitude, attention, memory) and attitudes (mood); academic behaviors (on-task behavior, concentration); and academic achievement (standardized test scores, reading literacy scores, or math fluency scores). Eight of the nine studies found positive associations between classroom-based physical activity and indicators of cognitive skills and attitudes, academic behavior, and academic achievement; none of the studies found negative associations.

### 4) Extracurricular Physical Activity Studies

Nineteen studies (reported in 14 articles) focused specifically on the relationship between academic performance and activities organized through school that occur outside of the regular school day. These activities included participation in school sports (interscholastic sports and other team or individual sports) as well as other after-school physical activity programs. All 19 studies examining the relationships between participation in extracurricular physical activities and academic performance found one or more positive associations.

## Strengths and Limitations

This review has a number of strengths. It involved a systematic process for locating, reviewing, and coding the studies. Studies were obtained using an extensive array of search terms and international databases and were reviewed by multiple trained coders. The studies cover a broad array of contexts in which youth participate in school-based physical activities and span a period of 23 years. Furthermore, a majority (64%) of studies included in the review were intervention studies, and a majority (76%) were longitudinal.

The breadth of the review, however, is a limitation. All studies meeting the established review criteria were included and treated equally, regardless of the study characteristics (e.g., design, sample size). The studies were not ranked, weighted, or grouped according to their strengths and limitations. The breadth of the review, while revealing a variety of study designs, measures, and populations, often made comparisons and summaries difficult. As a result, conclusions are intentionally broad.

## Implications for Policy

There are a number of policy implications stemming from this review:

- There is substantial evidence that physical activity can help improve academic achievement, including grades and standardized test scores.

- The articles in this review suggest that physical activity can have an impact on cognitive skills and attitudes and academic behavior, all of which are important components of improved academic performance. These include enhanced concentration and attention as well as improved classroom behavior.

- Increasing or maintaining time dedicated to physical education may help, and does not appear to adversely impact, academic performance.

# Implications for Schools

The results of this review support several strategies that schools can use to help students meet national physical activity recommendations without detracting from academic performance:

- **School-based physical education:** To maximize the potential benefits of student participation in physical education class, schools and physical education teachers can consider increasing the amount of time students spend in physical education or adding components to increase the quality of physical education class. Articles in the review examined increased physical education time (achieved by increasing the number of days physical education was provided each week or lengthening class time) and/or improved quality of physical education (achieved through strategies such as using trained instructors and increasing the amount of active time during physical education class).

- **Recess:** School boards, superintendents, principals, and teachers can feel confident that providing recess to students on a regular basis may benefit academic behaviors, while also facilitating social development and contributing to overall physical activity and its associated health benefits. There was no evidence that time spent in recess had a negative association with cognitive skills, attitudes, or academic behavior.

- **Classroom-based physical activity:** Classroom teachers can incorporate movement activities and physical activity breaks into the classroom setting that may improve student performance and the classroom environment. Most interventions reviewed here used short breaks (5–20 minutes) that required little or no teacher preparation, special equipment, or resources.

- **Extracurricular physical activities:** The evidence suggests that superintendents, principals, and athletic directors can develop or continue school-based sports programs without concern that these activities have a detrimental impact on students' academic performance. School administrators and teachers also can encourage after-school organizations, clubs, student groups, and parent groups to incorporate physical activities into their programs and events.

# INTRODUCTION

When children and adolescents participate in at least 60 minutes of physical activity every day, multiple health benefits accrue.[1,2] Regular physical activity builds healthy bones and muscles, improves muscular strength and endurance, reduces the risk for developing chronic disease risk factors, improves self-esteem, and reduces stress and anxiety.[1] Beyond these known health effects, physical activity may also have beneficial influences on academic performance.

Children and adolescents engage in different types of physical activity, depending on age and access to programs and equipment in their schools and communities. Elementary school-aged children typically engage in free play, running and chasing games, jumping rope, and age-appropriate sports—activities that are aligned with the development of fundamental motor skills. The development of complex motor skills enables adolescents to engage in active recreation (e.g., canoeing, skiing, rollerblading), resistance exercises with weights or weight machines, individual sports (e.g., running, bicycling), and team sports (e.g., basketball, baseball).[1,3] Most youth, however, do not engage in the recommended level of physical activity. For example,

only 17.1% of U.S. high school students meet current recommendations for physical activity (CDC, unpublished data, 2009).

Schools, which serve nearly 56 million youth in the United States, provide a unique venue for youth to meet the physical activity recommendations.[4] At the same time, schools face increasing challenges in allocating time for physical education and physical activity during the school day. Many schools are attempting to increase instructional time for mathematics, English, and science in an effort to improve standards-based test scores.[5] As a result, physical education classes, recess, and other physical activity breaks often are decreased or eliminated during the school day. This is evidenced by data from both students and schools. For example, in 2007 only 53.6% of U.S. high school students reported that they attended physical education class on 1 or more days in an average week at school, and fewer (30%) reported participating in physical education classes daily.[6] Similarly, in 2006 only 4% of elementary schools, 8% of middle schools, and 2% of high schools in the United States provided daily physical education or its equivalent for all students in all grades.[7] Furthermore, in 2006 only 57% of all school districts required that elementary schools provide students with regularly scheduled recess. As for physical activity outside of physical education and recess, during the school day, 16% of school districts required elementary schools, 10% required middle schools, and 4% required high schools to provide regular physical activity breaks.[7]

In addition to school-day opportunities, youth also have opportunities to participate in physical activity through extracurricular physical activities (e.g., school sports, recreation, other teams), which may be available through schools, communities, and/or after-school programs.[8] Seventy-six percent of 6- to 12-year-olds reported participating in some sports in 1997,[9] and in 2007, 56% of high school students reported playing on one or more sports teams organized by their school or community in the previous 12 months.[6]

There is a growing body of research focused on the association between school-based physical activity, including physical education, and academic

## Defining Academic Performance

*In this review, academic performance is used broadly to describe different factors that may influence student success in school. These factors fall into three primary areas:*

- *Cognitive Skills and Attitudes (e.g., attention/concentration, memory, verbal ability).*

- *Academic Behaviors (e.g., conduct, attendance, time on task, homework completion).*

- *Academic Achievement (e.g., standardized test scores, grades).*

performance among school-aged youth.[3,10-16] This developing literature suggests that physical activity may have an impact on academic performance through a variety of direct and indirect physiological, cognitive, emotional, and learning mechanisms.[12,17,18] Research on brain development indicates that cognitive development occurs in tandem with motor ability.[19]

Several review articles also have examined the connections between physical activity and academic behavior and achievement. Sibley and Etnier[12] conducted a meta-analysis of published studies relating physical activity and cognition in youth. Two additional reviews described the evidence for relationships between physical activity, brain physiology, cognition, emotion, and academic achievement among children, drawing from studies of humans and other animals across the lifespan.[14,20] Finally, two other reviews summarized select peer-reviewed research on the relationship between physical activity and academic performance, with an emphasis on school settings and policies.[15,16]

Research also has explored the relationships among physical education and physical activity, fitness levels and motor skill development, and academic performance. For example, several studies have shown a positive relationship between increased physical fitness levels and academic achievement[10,21-27] as well as fitness levels and measures of cognitive skills and attitudes.[28] In addition, other studies have shown that improved motor skill levels are positively related to improvements in academic achievement[29-31] and measures of cognitive skills and attitudes.[32-34]

To extend the understanding of these connections, this review offers a broad examination of the literature on a range of physical activity contexts, including physical education classes, recess, classroom-based physical activity breaks outside of physical education class and recess, and extracurricular physical activity, thereby providing a tool to inform program and policy efforts for education and health professionals. The purpose of this report is to synthesize the scientific literature that has examined the association between school-based physical activity, including physical education, and academic performance, including indicators of cognitive skills and attitudes, academic behaviors, and academic achievement.

## How Physical Activity Affects the Brain[16][18]

*Cognitive skills and motor skills appear to develop through a dynamic interaction. Research has shown that physical movement can affect the brain's physiology by increasing*

- *Cerebral capillary growth.*

- *Blood flow.*

- *Oxygenation.*

- *Production of neurotrophins.*

- *Growth of nerve cells in the hippocampus (center of learning and memory).*

- *Neurotransmitter levels.*

- *Development of nerve connections.*

- *Density of neural network.*

- *Brain tissue volume.*

*These physiological changes may be associated with*

- *Improved attention.*

- *Improved information processing, storage, and retrieval.*

- *Enhanced coping.*

- *Enhanced positive affect.*

- *Reduced sensations of cravings and pain.*

# METHODS

## Conceptual Definitions

The research on this topic suggests that physical activity can be related to many different aspects of academic performance (e.g., attention, on-task behavior, grade-point average [GPA]), and as a result, the existing literature examines a wide range of variables. In this report, those variables are organized into three categories: 1) cognitive skills and attitudes, 2) academic behaviors, and 3) academic achievement. The three categories, as well as other important terms used in this report, are defined below.

**Academic Performance:** In this review, academic performance is used broadly to describe different factors that may influence student success in school. These factors are grouped into three primary areas:

### 1) Cognitive Skills and Attitudes

Cognitive skills and attitudes include both basic cognitive abilities, such as executive functioning, attention, memory, verbal comprehension, and information processing, as well as attitudes and beliefs that influence academic performance, such as motivation, self-concept, satisfaction, and school connectedness. Studies used a range of measures to define and describe these constructs.

### 2) Academic Behaviors

Academic behaviors include a range of behaviors that may have an impact on students' academic performance. Common indicators include on-task behavior, organization, planning, attendance, scheduling, and impulse control. Studies used a range of measures to define and describe these constructs.

### 3) Academic Achievement

Academic achievement includes standardized test scores in subject areas such as reading, math, and language arts; GPAs; classroom test scores; and other formal assessments.

**Physical Education:** Physical education, as defined by the National Association for Sport and Physical Education (NASPE), is a curricular area offered in K–12 schools that provides students with instruction on physical activity, health-related fitness, physical competence, and cognitive understanding about physical activity, thereby enabling students to adopt healthy and physically active lifestyles.[35] A high-quality physical education program enables students to develop motor skills, understand movement concepts, participate in regular physical activity, maintain healthy fitness levels, develop responsible personal and social behavior, and value physical activity.[35]

**Recess:** Recess is a time during the school day that provides children with the opportunity for active, unstructured or structured, free play.

**Physical Activity:** Physical activity is defined as any bodily movement produced by the contraction of skeletal muscle that increases energy expenditure above a resting level.[1] Physical activity can be repetitive, structured, and planned movement (e.g., a fitness class or recreational activity such as hiking); leisurely (e.g., gardening); sports-focused (e.g., basketball, volleyball); work-related (e.g., lifting and moving boxes); or transportation-related (e.g., walking to school). The studies in this review included a range of ways to capture the frequency, intensity, duration, and type of students' physical activity.

**Physiology:** In this report, physiology includes indicators of structural or functional changes in the brain and body. Studies most often reported measures of physical fitness, motor skills, and body composition from this construct.

## Inclusion Criteria

The following criteria were used to identify published studies for inclusion in this review. Studies had to

- Be published in English.

- Present original data.

- Be published between 1985 and October 2008.*

- Focus on school-aged children aged 5–18 years.

- Include clear measures of physical education and/or physical activity, such as
  - Physical education class.
  - Recess.
  - Classroom-based physical activity (outside of physical education and recess).
  - Extracurricular physical activities (including school sports and other teams).

- Measure academic performance (cognitive skills and attitudes, academic behaviors, and academic achievement) using one or more educational or behavioral outcomes. Examples include
  - Graduation or dropout rates (n=2).
  - Performance on standardized tests (n=17).
  - Academic grades/GPA (n=9).
  - Years of school completed (n=1).
  - Time on task (n=3).
  - Concentration or attentiveness in educational settings (n=7).
  - Attendance (n=3).
  - Disciplinary problems (n=6).
  - School connectedness† (n=2).

Studies were excluded if they did not meet the above criteria or if they focused solely on sedentary lifestyle variables, overweight status, or media use rather than physical activity. Studies also were excluded if they focused exclusively on the relationship between academic performance and fitness test scores rather than physical activity itself. Review articles, meta-analyses, and unpublished studies were excluded from the coding and analysis portion of this review, although their reference lists were used to identify original research to be reviewed for inclusion.

---

* Articles published between October 2008 and the publication date that met the inclusion criteria and made a notable contribution to the field may have been included in the review based on expert recommendations.

† School connectedness refers to students' belief that adults and peers in the school care about their learning as well as about them as individuals.[36]

# Identification of Studies that Met the Inclusion Criteria

Studies were identified through a search of nine electronic databases (ERIC, Expanded Academic Index ASAP, Google Scholar, PsycNET®, PubMed, ScienceDirect®, Sociological Abstracts, SportDiscus™), and the Cumulative Index to Nursing and Allied Health Literature (CINAHL®) using a pre-established set of search terms that included both physical activity and academic-related terms (see Appendix A). Additional studies also were located from reference lists of the identified articles.

# Classification of Studies

The search yielded 406 articles (see Figure 1). Two trained researchers examined each article to determine its match with the inclusion criteria; it was then classified as "included for review" or "excluded from review." When the match was unclear, articles were temporarily classified as "possible inclusion" before being reviewed by two additional researchers for final classification. Initially, 50 articles were identified for inclusion. Four of those articles were later excluded because they lacked clarity necessary to categorize them appropriately for the review. For example, one article examining movement lacked sufficient information to determine whether the movement should be classified as physical activity; another article lacked a clear academic performance variable. The other two articles lacked clarity in descriptions of analyses and testing of research questions that was necessary for categorization. A fifth article was excluded because of its focus on elite athletes rather than a general student population. Two additional articles that examined associations between participation in a sports-based interdisciplinary curriculum and academic grades were excluded because of insufficient detail about the physical activity participation levels of students and the subsequent lack of fit into the review categories.

A total of 363 articles were excluded. Reasons for exclusion were failure to include an appropriate measure of physical activity (n=103), academic achievement (n=40), or both physical activity and academic achievement (n=25); classification as a review or meta-analysis (n=82); inclusion of participants outside the

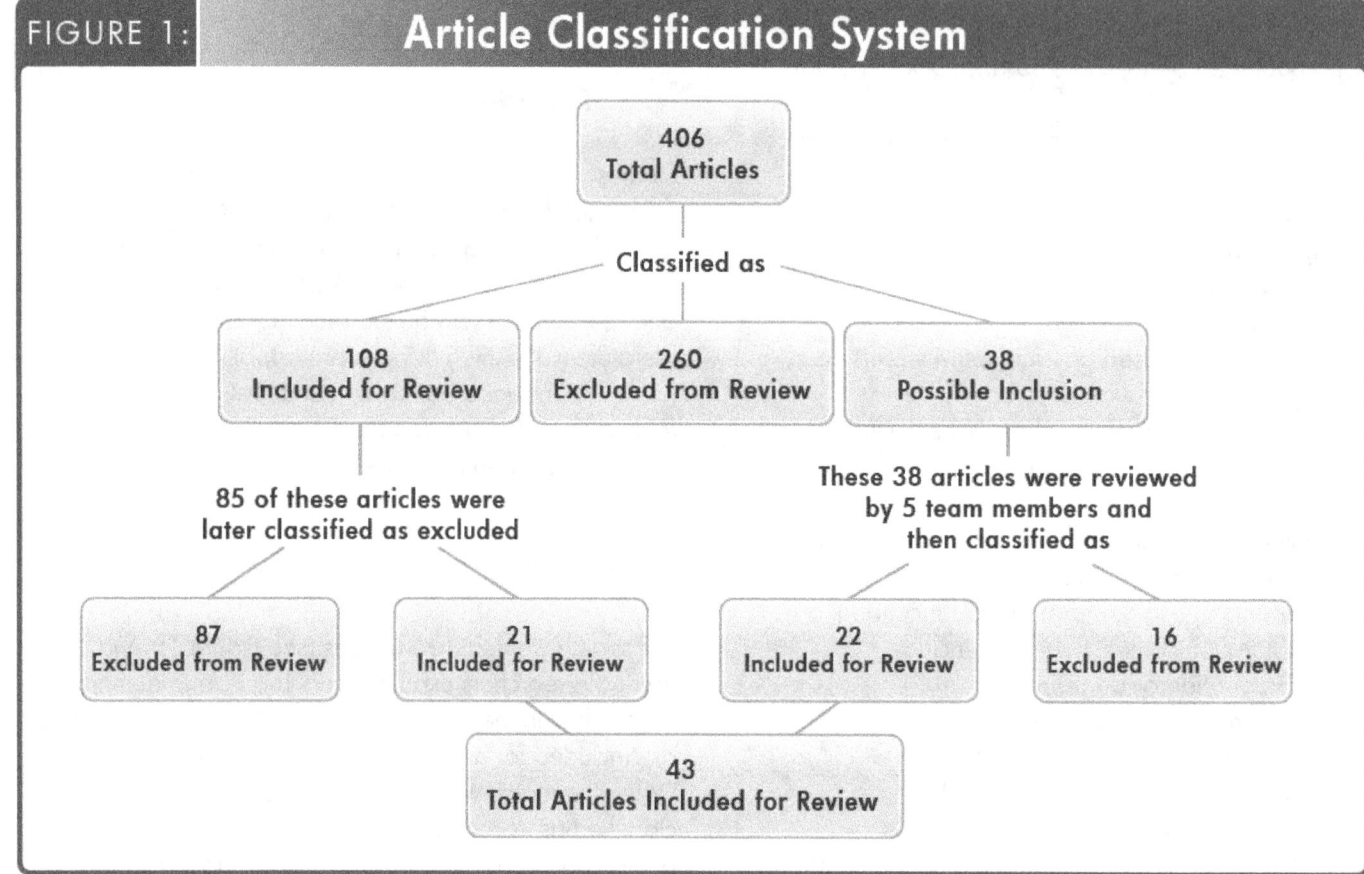

**FIGURE 1: Article Classification System**

406
Total Articles

Classified as

108
Included for Review

260
Excluded from Review

38
Possible Inclusion

85 of these articles were
later classified as excluded

These 38 articles were reviewed
by 5 team members and
then classified as

87
Excluded from Review

21
Included for Review

22
Included for Review

16
Excluded from Review

43
Total Articles Included for Review

age range of interest (n=58); inability to obtain full text of the study (n=49); and a publication date outside the inclusion range (n=6).

Overall, 43 articles (describing 50 unique studies) met the inclusion criteria and were read, abstracted, and coded for this synthesis. Two articles in this review presented findings from more than one study that met inclusion criteria; one article described three studies,[37] and the other reported six.[2]

## Study Coding Process

The coding method for this report is similar to that of several prominent literature reviews in the public health field.[38-40] A team of eight trained reviewers read and coded the 43 articles using a standard coding protocol (see Appendix B). When multiple studies were presented in a single article, this information was noted in the coding, but the studies remained grouped by article. The coding protocol involved abstracting information from the studies and entering it into a Microsoft Access® database.

Whenever possible, information was abstracted directly from articles as stated by authors. The following information was abstracted: purpose, research questions, study design, sampling, sample characteristics, setting, theory, intervention, methods, analytic strategy, results, limitations, study focus, and additional comments. For this review, study designs were classified as experimental, quasi-experimental, descriptive, or case studies (study designs are defined in Appendix C); data collection methods and time points were noted as described. Studies that lacked details regarding any field of interest were coded as "information not provided."

To ensure consistency in coding, approximately 17% of all articles were double-coded by a reviewer and a senior coder. A team of article reviewers met regularly during the coding process to discuss and resolve issues associated with coding. A system was established for handling coding questions and concerns. Senior team members resolved and verified issues as they arose.

A brief summary profile of each study was then created (see Appendices D–G). A list of the studies classified as using quasi-experimental or experimental designs is provided at the beginning of each of these appendices. These summaries were e-mailed to the studies' corresponding authors for review and verification. Authors not responding within the initial timeline received a second request for review. Seventy-two percent of the authors (31 of 43) reviewed their summaries. Author edits and suggestions were incorporated where applicable.

## Data Analysis

Coded data from the articles were used to categorize and organize studies first by their physical activity context and then by outcome, cohort, sampling groups, and date published. The individual studies were identified (in the instances where articles described more than one study), and all reviewed studies were treated equally, regardless of study characteristics or design. Although meta-analysis was considered as a method to analyze data in this review, the small number and heterogeneity of studies precluded use of that method. Therefore, descriptive literature synthesis was conducted. In this report, the results describe the types of associations or relationships reported in the studies. When positive or negative associations are described in the Results section below, they refer to findings that the study authors reported as reaching statistical significance ($p \leq 0.05$).

# RESULTS

This review examines the findings of 43 articles (reflective of 50 studies total) that explored the relationship between physical activity and/or physical education and academic performance. Each study was categorized in one of four physical activity context areas: 1) school-based physical education; 2) recess; 3) classroom-based physical activity (outside of physical education and recess); and 4) extracurricular physical activity.

*School-based physical education* as a context category encompassed all studies that were explicitly set in physical education class or consisted of a school-based course or curriculum that addressed primary aspects of physical education. This category included activities conducted in physical education class but did not exclude curricula with components that extended beyond formal physical education. Typically, studies in this category examined the impact of increasing the amount of time students spent in physical education class or manipulating the types of activities conducted with students.

*Recess* studies explored the relationship between academic performance and recess during the school day in elementary schools. Recess is typically 10–15 minutes or longer of unstructured free play that may occur as a break during the school day or in association with lunch.

*Classroom-based physical activity* as a context category included studies that were classroom-based but were not physical education class or recess. In general, these studies explored short physical activity breaks (5–20 minutes) or ways to introduce physical activity into learning activities that were either designed to promote learning through physical activity or provide students with a pure physical activity break. These interventions are relatively easy and inexpensive for a teacher to incorporate into the classroom.

*Extracurricular physical activity* as a context category encompassed studies that focused specifically on the relationships between activities organized through school that occur outside of the regular school day. This category included participation in school sports (interscholastic sports and other teams) as well as other after-school physical activity programs.

## Results at a Glance

*For the 43 articles reviewed,*

- *A total of 251 associations between physical activity and academic performance were measured.*

- *The most commonly measured indicator of academic performance was cognitive skills and attitudes (112 of the 251 associations tested).*

- *More than half (50.5%) of all associations tested were positive.*

- *Positive associations were found across measures of academic achievement, academic behavior, and cognitive skills and attitudes.*

- *There were only four negative associations, accounting for 1.5% of all associations tested.*

Of all 50 studies in the review, almost two-thirds (62%) focused on youth physical activity experiences through school-based physical education, during recess, or in the classroom; the remaining studies (38%) examined extracurricular physical activity (see Table 1). Slightly more than half (54%) of the articles focused exclusively on students in secondary school settings; 44% included studies conducted with elementary students; and 2% included both elementary and secondary grade levels. The scope and research designs varied as well. Most studies were descriptive (44%) or quasi-experimental (34%) in nature, and the majority (76%) reported longitudinal data. Most studies (80%) were conducted during the school day, and about two-thirds (64%) included a physical education or physical activity intervention. Finally, the majority (68%) of studies were conducted in the United States; overall, studies were conducted in nine countries other than the United States.

For ease of review, the results are presented here by physical activity context. Within each context, results are described by study focus (intervention or nonintervention) and by the type of results.

Each results subsection also includes a summary table that shows the number of associations (total, positive, negative, and no association) for all the studies reviewed in that context area. Results with $p$ values less than 0.05 are considered statistically significant in this report. Qualitative and descriptive studies that did not include significance testing are described in the text of this report, but not in the outcome counts. Associations are displayed by type of academic performance outcome measured: cognitive skills and attitudes, academic behavior, or academic achievement.

## Table 1: Summary Characteristics of Reviewed Studies

| Characteristics of Studies | Number of Studies (N=50) | Number of Studies that Included Academic Achievement Measure* | | |
| | | Academic Achievement | Academic Behavior | Cognitive Skills and Attitudes |
|---|---|---|---|---|
| **Physical Activity Context** | | | | |
| Physical education class | 14 | 10 | 3 | 7 |
| Recess | 8 | 0 | 3 | 5 |
| Classroom based | 9 | 6 | 1 | 5 |
| Extracurricular physical activity | 19 | 16 | 9 | 14 |
| **Study Design** | | | | |
| Experimental | 11 | 8 | 3 | 6 |
| Quasi-experimental | 17 | 6 | 4 | 12 |
| Descriptive | 22 | 17 | 11 | 11 |
| **Data Collection Design** | | | | |
| Cross-sectional | 12 | 8 | 3 | 5 |
| Longitudinal | 38 | 27 | 15 | 26 |
| **Intervention** | | | | |
| Intervention | 32 | 20 | 12 | 23 |
| Nonintervention | 18 | 15 | 6 | 8 |
| **Setting†** | | | | |
| School day | 40 | 26 | 12 | 22 |
| After school | 6 | 5 | 2 | 5 |
| Community | 3 | 3 | 3 | 3 |
| Household | 2 | 2 | 1 | 2 |
| **Student Sample Educational Level** | | | | |
| Primary | 22 | 12 | 6 | 11 |
| Secondary | 27 | 23 | 11 | 19 |
| Cross level | 1 | 0 | 1 | 1 |
| **Country** | | | | |
| United States | 34 | 23 | 16 | 21 |
| International | 16 | 12 | 2 | 10 |

* Studies often included more than one type of measure; thus, the number of studies that include these different academic performance measures may exceed the total number of studies in any given category.

† Some studies included more than one setting; therefore, the total number of studies by setting exceeds 50.

# School-Based Physical Education Studies

Fourteen studies (reported in 14 articles) examined the relationship between school-based physical education and academic performance (see Figure 2, and Tables 2a and 2b). Most (n=10) described intervention studies and assessed the impact of an intervention on a range of outcomes. The remaining four were descriptive and examined the relationships between physical education and academic measures. Appendix D includes summary profiles for each of the articles reviewed in this section.

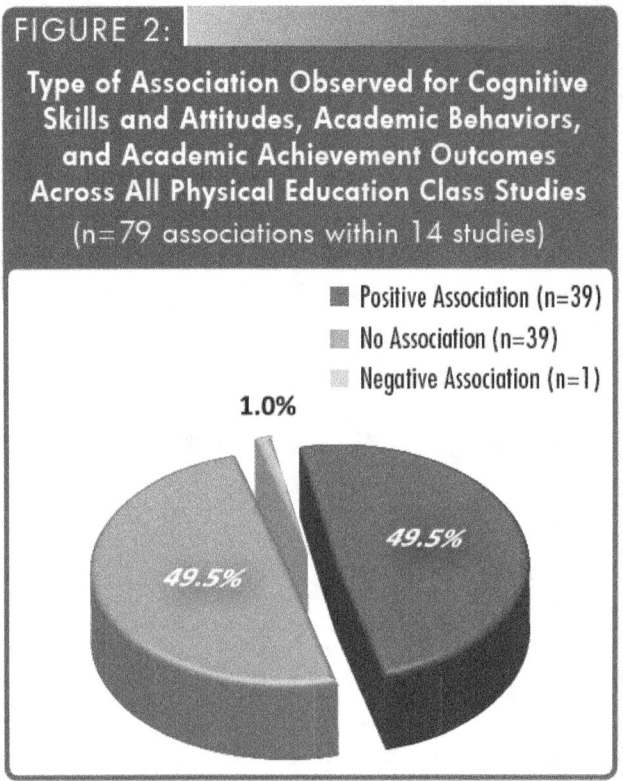

## FIGURE 2:

**Type of Association Observed for Cognitive Skills and Attitudes, Academic Behaviors, and Academic Achievement Outcomes Across All Physical Education Class Studies** (n=79 associations within 14 studies)

- ■ Positive Association (n=39)
- ■ No Association (n=39)
- ■ Negative Association (n=1)

1.0%

49.5%

49.5%

**Intervention Studies.** In general, the intervention studies (three implemented in the United States and seven in other countries) examined how differences in physical education affected academic performance. Six studies[41-46] examined increasing the amount of physical education or the level of physical activity intensity in physical education class and comparing students' academic performance by intervention condition (e.g., physical education two times per week versus daily physical education, or physical education for 20 minutes versus physical education for 30 or 40 minutes, or the intensity of physical activity during physical education).

### School-Based Physical Education Studies: Highlights

- *Eleven of 14 studies found one or more positive associations between physical education and indicators of cognitive skills and attitudes, academic behavior, and/or academic achievement.*

- *Overall, increased time in physical education appears to have a positive relationship or no relationship with academic achievement.*

- *Increased time in physical education does not appear to have a negative relationship with academic achievement.*

Two studies examined strategies for improving the quality of physical education: one focused on implementation by trained instructors of a curriculum that promotes greater amounts of moderate and vigorous physical activity in students, and the other implemented multiple strategies such as focusing on students' personal goal setting, emphasizing opportunities for active participation by all students, and maximizing active use of class time.[47,48] The remaining two studies examined the relationship between increasing the emphasis on different types of activities (i.e., aerobic exercise, coordinative exercise) and aspects of academic performance.[49,50]

Collectively, the studies were conducted across a broad range of grade levels, representing elementary, middle, and high schools. Seven studies employed an experimental design, and three reported data from quasi-experimental designs. Most studies involved short-term follow-up (e.g., immediate or 3-month delay). Sallis and colleagues[48] and Ericsson[43] both followed youth for approximately 3 years.

Finally, the studies assessed a range of indicators of academic performance, including cognitive skills (e.g., concentration and creativity), attitudes (e.g., self-esteem and motivation), academic behaviors (e.g., conduct), and/or academic achievement (e.g., standardized test scores and GPA).

Results varied across the 10 intervention studies, with most (8 of 10) showing one or more positive associations. Two studies showed all or mostly positive associations between physical education and cognitive skills and attitudes or academic achievement. Specifically, Ericsson[43] found that extending physical education (from 2 days per week to daily) was associated positively with academic achievement (math, reading, and writing test scores). That study also noted positive associations

for attention, an indicator of cognitive functioning, although the relationships dissipated over time. Budde and colleagues[49] found that coordination exercises (i.e., exercises that require the body to balance, react, adjust, and/or differentiate) were more beneficial than normal sport lessons in boosting cognitive functioning (specifically, concentration and attention).

Six studies reported more mixed conclusions. Five found a mixture of positive and nonsignificant associations.[41,42,44,47,50] For example, Dwyer and colleagues[42] compared academic achievement and classroom behavior across three intervention conditions

## Table 2a: School-Based Physical Education Intervention Studies: Summary of the Outcomes of Cognitive Skills and Attitudes, Academic Behaviors, and Academic Achievement

| Variables in Physical Education Intervention Studies (N=10 Studies)* | Total # of Performance Outcomes Across the 10 Intervention Studies | Type of Relationship Observed Between Physical Education Class and Academic Performance | | |
|---|---|---|---|---|
| | | Positive | None | Negative |
| **Cognitive Skills and Attitudes (N=7 Studies)** | **24** | **12** | **12** | **0** |
| Attention/concentration | 5 | 3 | 2 | 0 |
| Self-esteem | 1 | 1 | 0 | 0 |
| Creativity | 1 | 1 | 0 | 0 |
| Perception of academic or intellectual competence/self-concept | 8 | 3 | 5 | 0 |
| Perceptual motor ability | 1 | 0 | 1 | 0 |
| Planning ability | 1 | 0 | 1 | 0 |
| Perceived self-concept | 2 | 1 | 1 | 0 |
| Impulse control | 3 | 2 | 1 | 0 |
| Life satisfaction | 1 | 1 | 0 | 0 |
| Attitude towards school | 1 | 0 | 1 | 0 |
| **Academic Behavior (N=3 Studies)** | **7** | **2** | **5** | **0** |
| Conduct | 7 | 2 | 5 | 0 |
| **Academic Achievement (N=6 Studies)** | **21** | **11** | **9** | **1** |
| Achievement test scores (e.g., math, reading, language arts) | 19 | 10 | 8 | 1 |
| Grades/grade point average | 2 | 1 | 1 | 0 |
| **Total** | **52** | **25** | **26** | **1** |

* Studies may have measured the relationship between physical education class and academic performance in more than one way (e.g., measured the association between physical education class and standardized test scores, attendance, motivation, and perceived academic potential). Individual studies in this section measured between 1 and 8 different outcomes and may be represented in multiple cells of the table.

(fitness group: 75 minutes of activity daily, with an emphasis on intensity of activities; skill group: 75 minutes of activity daily with no focus on intensity; and control group: three 30-minute periods of physical education per week). They found no differences in academic achievement across the three intervention conditions, despite the fact that students in the fitness and skill groups actually had less classroom teaching time to accommodate the increase in time for physical education. They also found that classroom behavior improved for students in the skill and fitness intervention conditions. The sixth study found four positive and three nonsignificant associations, as well as one negative relationship.[48] Sallis and colleagues[48] examined an intensive 2-year health-related physical education program that was taught by trained classroom teachers or physical education specialists and was designed to increase students' physical activity levels. They found that the SPARK program taught by trained teachers had a positive impact on reading, language, and basic battery standardized test scores, but had no significant impact on math. When taught by physical education specialists, students in the SPARK program scored better than students not enrolled in SPARK on reading, but lower on language and about the same in math.

Finally, two studies found no associations between physical education and indicators of academic performance. These studies examined the relationship between the frequency of physical education and either cognitive skills and attitudes[46] or academic

achievement.[45] Raviv and Low[46] found that physical education did not reduce concentration, contrary to the beliefs of some teachers in their study. Pollatschek and O'Hagan[45] found that the frequency of physical education participation (daily versus twice a week) was not associated with students' standardized math and reading test scores or affect towards school; similar results were found for boys and girls.

Collectively, the results of these studies suggest that physical education may have favorable associations with students' cognitive skills and attitudes and their academic achievement, but the relationships are not universal and vary by outcome studied. Furthermore, increasing time for physical education does not appear to have negative associations with academic achievement.

**Nonintervention Studies.** The four nonintervention studies (two conducted in the United States and two in other countries) examined associations between physical education and academic performance using cross-sectional designs (n=3) or secondary analyses of an existing longitudinal data set (n=1). Three of the four studies were conducted at the elementary or middle school level; the fourth study was completed with high school students. All studies used standardized tests to assess academic achievement. Results were either positive or neutral. Three of the studies found positive associations between time spent in physical education or skills learned in physical education and indicators of academic achievement. As an example, one study[51]

## Table 2b: School-Based Physical Education Nonintervention Studies: Summary of the Outcomes of Academic Achievement

| Variables in Physical Education Nonintervention Studies (N=4 Studies)* | Total # of Performance Outcomes Across the 4 Nonintervention Studies | Type of Relationship Observed Between Physical Education Class and Academic Performance | | |
| --- | --- | --- | --- | --- |
| | | Positive | None | Negative |
| **Academic Achievement (N=4 Studies)** | **27** | **14** | **13** | **0** |
| Achievement test scores (e.g., math, reading, language arts) | 27 | 14 | 13 | 0 |
| **Total** | **27** | **14** | **13** | **0** |

* Studies may have measured the relationship between physical education class and academic performance in more than one way (e.g., measured the association between physical education class and multiple subjects in standardized test scores). Individual studies in this section measured between 2 and 14 different outcomes and may be represented in multiple cells of the table.

noted a positive association between standardized English language arts test scores and time spent in physical education but found no such association for math scores. Another study[52] found small but significant associations between physical education and academic achievement in math and reading for girls who had more physical education (70–300 minutes per week) compared with those getting lower amounts (0–35 minutes per week); none of the associations were significant for boys. Dexter[53] found a combination of positive associations and no association between performance on sports learned in physical education and an average of math and English test scores and grades, depending on the sport; results were similar for boys and girls. The remaining study found no significant associations between physical education and academic performance on state literacy and numeracy tests.[54] There were no negative associations between physical education and indicators of academic performance across these four studies. Consistent with the results of the physical education intervention studies, the data from these four studies suggest physical education has some positive associations with academic outcomes, but these results vary by outcome.

**Strengths and Limitations of Methods.** This collection of studies has a number of strengths as well as limitations. The studies were conducted across a range of grade levels and used a broad array of indicators related to cognitive skills, attitudes, and academic achievement. Furthermore, nearly half featured experimental designs, and half explored associations by gender. Several limitations were noted by the authors of the studies, including small samples or samples with potential biases that may affect the generalizability of the results (e.g., university research/laboratory school populations or affluent populations). Several authors acknowledged measurement issues, such as limited follow-up, not assessing precursors of academic achievement (e.g., concentration, memory, or classroom behavior), or failing to collect data on socioeconomic status (SES) and other potentially important background variables. Finally, authors of intervention studies also noted implementation limits, such as unequal participation in the intervention or lack of data on implementation quality. Many of the studies did not report data on the racial/ethnic characteristics of their samples, and only one examined results by racial/ethnic subgroups.

### Recess Studies: Highlights

- *All eight studies found one or more positive associations between recess and indicators of cognitive skills, attitudes, and academic behavior.*

- *Time spent in recess appears to have a positive relationship or no relationship with children's attention, concentration, and/or on-task classroom behavior.*

## Recess Studies

Eight studies (reported in six articles) examined the relationship between school recess, cognitive skills, attitudes, and/or academic behavior (see Figure 3, and Tables 3a and 3b). Six of the studies tested an intervention to examine how recess impacts these indicators of academic performance. The other two descriptive, nonintervention studies explored the relationships between recess and school adjustment or classroom behavior. Appendix E includes summary profiles for each of the articles reviewed in this section.

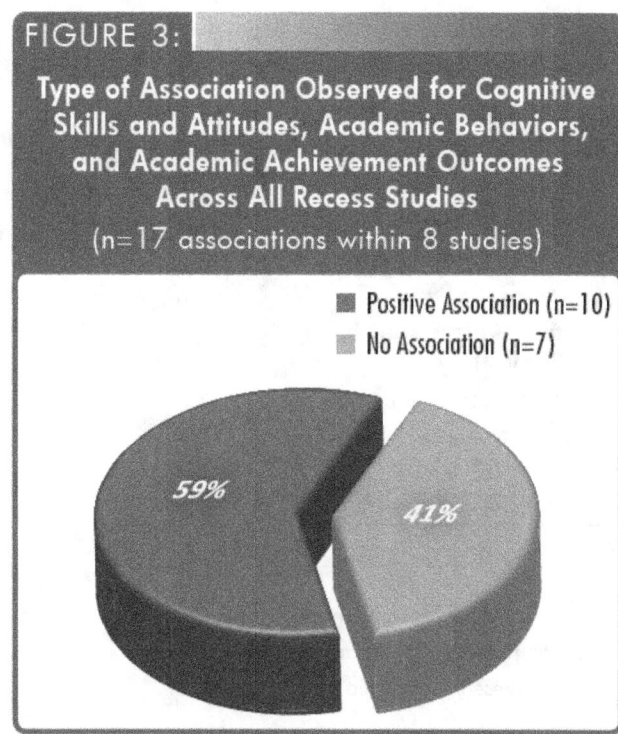

FIGURE 3:

**Type of Association Observed for Cognitive Skills and Attitudes, Academic Behaviors, and Academic Achievement Outcomes Across All Recess Studies**
(n=17 associations within 8 studies)

- Positive Association (n=10)
- No Association (n=7)

59%

41%

**Intervention Studies.** The six intervention studies (all implemented in the United States) examined the relationship between recess, or increased physical activity during recess, and cognitive skills (attention or concentration) and academic behavior (on-task behavior). All of these studies were conducted in elementary schools with students in kindergarten through fourth grade, and all six employed an experimental or quasi-experimental design.[37,55-57] Most used trained observers to collect data on classroom and recess behaviors, with multiple observation points. The data collection follow-up period ranged from 0 to 4 months following baseline. The interventions involved the introduction of recess into the daily school schedule or manipulating the timing of recess (e.g., holding recess after varying lengths of class time).

Results across these six studies showed positive outcomes or no association. Three studies reported all positive associations between more physical activity at recess and classroom behaviors.[55-57] Specifically, Caterino and Polak[55] found that fourth-grade students who participated in directed physical activity during recess (stretching and aerobic walking) had significantly higher concentration scores than those students who sat quietly in the library during recess. Both studies that measured academic behavior found a positive relationship between recess and on-task behavior. Jarrett and colleagues[56] observed that children were less fidgety, less listless, more focused,

and more on task when they had recess compared with when they did not have recess. Pellegrini and Davis[57] found that students who engaged in physical activity (as opposed to sedentary behavior) during recess fidgeted less in the classroom after recess.

The three intervention studies by Pellegrini and colleagues[37] reported both positive and nonsignificant associations. These studies examined the relationships between the timing of recess (i.e., recess after 2.5 hours versus 3 hours of classroom time) and students' behaviors during recess and students' classroom behaviors before and after recess. Investigators found that students' attention rates were lower after longer periods of classroom work without a break than after shorter periods. They also found that, in general, students' attention was better after recess than before. Finally, they found that the type of behavior during recess did not affect classroom attention after recess for any grade or gender groups.

**Nonintervention Studies.** One of the two nonintervention recess studies[58] explored the impact of the frequency of recess on teacher reports of classroom behavior in a very large sample (n=11,529); the other[59] explored the impact of recess on observations of individual students' cognitive and emotional adjustment to school within one school (n=77). Barros, Silver, and Stein[58] found that overall classroom behavior (based on

## Table 3a: Recess Intervention Studies: Summary of the Outcomes of Cognitive Skills and Attitudes and Academic Behaviors

| Variables in Recess Intervention Studies (N=6 Studies)* | Total # of Performance Outcomes Across the 6 Intervention Studies | Type of Relationship Observed Between Recess and Academic Performance | | |
|---|---|---|---|---|
| | | Positive | None | Negative |
| **Cognitive Skills and Attitudes (N=4 Studies)** | **10** | **4** | **6** | **0** |
| Attention/concentration | 10 | 4 | 6 | 0 |
| **Academic Behavior (N=2 Studies)** | **4** | **4** | **0** | **0** |
| On-task behavior (not fidgeting) | 4 | 4 | 0 | 0 |
| **Total** | **14** | **8** | **6** | **0** |

* Studies may have measured the relationship between recess and academic performance in more than one way (e.g., measured the association between recess and attention and behavior). Individual studies in this section measured between 1 and 9 different outcomes and may be represented in multiple cells of the table.

## Table 3b: Recess Nonintervention Studies: Summary of the Outcomes of Cognitive Skills and Attitudes and Academic Behaviors

| Variables in Recess Nonintervention Studies (N=2 Studies)* | Total # of Performance Outcomes Across the 2 Nonintervention Studies | Type of Relationship Observed Between Recess and Academic Performance | | |
|---|---|---|---|---|
| | | Positive | None | Negative |
| **Cognitive Skills and Attitudes (N=1 Study)** | **2** | **1** | **1** | **0** |
| Perceptions of school adjustment | 2 | 1 | 1 | 0 |
| **Academic Behavior (N=1 Study)** | **1** | **1** | **0** | **0** |
| On-task behavior (not fidgeting) | 1 | 1 | 0 | 0 |
| **Total** | **3** | **2** | **1** | **0** |

* Studies may have measured the relationship between recess and academic performance in more than one way (e.g., measured the association between recess and perceptions of school adjustment and on-task behavior). Individual studies in this section measured between 1 and 2 different outcomes and may be represented in multiple cells of the table.

teacher ratings) was significantly better for students who had recess every day for at least 15 minutes than for those who did not. Exploration of the impact of recess on individual students showed a positive association with end-of-year social competence and perceptions of school adjustment for boys, but not for girls.[59]

**Strengths and Limitations of Methods.** These studies feature several strengths as well as a few notable limitations. Six of the eight studies used experimental or quasi-experimental designs, and most involved observations of student behaviors with multiple observation points (e.g., 6, 12, or 32 observations). The studies focused on elementary-level students, primarily because recess is most common at the elementary grade levels. Study authors reported a number of limitations including small sample sizes (range of 23–77 students in seven of the eight studies), and the inability in most of the studies to analyze data by SES, race/ethnicity, or other subgroups. In addition, the authors noted that classroom-level ratings of student behavior by the classroom teacher could be influenced by the teachers' perceptions of the benefits of recess.

## Classroom Physical Activity Studies

Nine studies (reported in nine articles) examined the relationship between classroom-based physical activity and academic performance (four implemented in the United States and five in other countries) (see Figure 4 and Table 4). All nine of the studies were interventions. Appendix F includes summary profiles for each of the articles reviewed in this section.

These studies examined how the introduction of brief physical activities in a classroom setting affected cognitive skills (e.g., aptitude, attention, memory); attitudes (e.g., mood); academic behaviors (e.g., on-task behavior, concentration); and academic achievement (e.g., standardized test scores, reading literacy scores, math fluency scores). The interventions involved the introduction of physical activities by trained teachers or facilitators into the classroom setting, with activities lasting 5–20 minutes per session. Physical activity sessions or breaks typically were delivered on a daily or regular basis. Intervention implementation periods spanned from 1 day to 16 months, with most lasting 2–3 months.

All but two of these studies were conducted with elementary school students in first through fifth grades; the others were conducted in a primary and secondary school in Sweden[60] and an urban middle school in the United States.[61] Five studies employed quasi-experimental designs,[60-64] three used experimental designs,[32,65-67] and one used a qualitative case-study design.[68] The data collection follow-up period ranged from 0 to 12 months after the intervention. Outcome measures most often included standardized aptitude and achievement tests and teacher or trained observer ratings of classroom behavior.

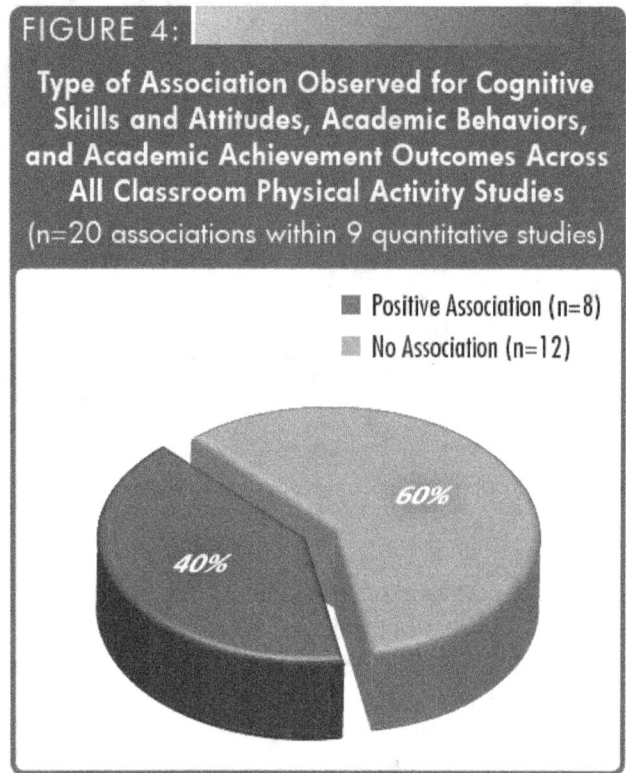

**FIGURE 4:**

**Type of Association Observed for Cognitive Skills and Attitudes, Academic Behaviors, and Academic Achievement Outcomes Across All Classroom Physical Activity Studies**
(n=20 associations within 9 quantitative studies)

■ Positive Association (n=8)
▨ No Association (n=12)

60%

40%

**Classroom Physical Activity Studies: Highlights**

• *Eight of the nine studies found positive associations between classroom-based physical activity and indicators of academic performance.*

• *One study examined gender effects and found no differences in outcomes by gender.*

Results across the nine intervention studies showed positive outcomes or no association. Four studies reported all positive associations between classroom physical activity and classroom behaviors and academic achievement.[60-63] Specifically, Della Valle and colleagues[61] found using movement with seventh-grade learners who had an active learning style enhanced their performance on a word recognition task. Maeda and Randall[62] reported that second-grade students exhibited greater concentration and demonstrated higher math fluency after engaging in brief movement breaks consisting of 5 minutes of vigorous exercise 1 hour after lunch. Similarly, Mahar et al.[63] observed greater frequency of verbal and motor behavior that followed class rules and was appropriate to the learning situation for third- and fourth-grade students whose teachers led them in daily 10-minute regimens of physical activities (e.g., jumping, rolling, hopping, twisting) during academic instruction. This relationship was especially strong among students who were least on task at baseline. Furthermore, Norlander and colleagues[60] found that teachers observed higher student concentration levels after daily stretching exercises.

Four intervention studies reported positive and nonsignificant associations.[64,66-68] Fredericks et al.[66] described improvements in spatial aptitude, reading skills, and math skills among first-grade students exposed to daily classroom exercises focused on the development of perceptual and sensory motor skills. However, there were no associations with other indicators of aptitude, such as perception, reasoning, memory, and verbal comprehension or emotional indicators. In their feasibility study, Lowden et al.[68] qualitatively described that students and teachers perceived that student exposure to *The Class Moves!®* program was positively related to improvements in on-task classroom behaviors and concentration. Teachers, however, did not feel they could relate the program to academic or cognitive achievement. Molloy[64] observed that students exposed to 5 minutes, but not 10 minutes, of aerobic exercise improved their arithmetic performance. Exposure to aerobic exercise was unrelated to observed on-task behavior (attention) for all but a small sample of hyperactive students. Uhrich and Swalm[67] found that daily sessions to develop motor skills (bimanual coordination) through a sport cup-stacking exercise were associated with improvements in reading comprehension but not reading decoding scores. These improvements were comparable for boys and girls.

The ninth intervention study found no relationship between an additional 15 minutes of daily classroom-based physical activity (skipping, dancing, and resistance exercises) in the context of a school-wide physical activity program and standardized achievement tests.[65] The classroom intervention lasted

## Table 4: Classroom Physical Activity Intervention Studies: Summary of the Outcomes of Cognitive Skills and Attitudes, Academic Behaviors, and Academic Achievement

| Variables in Classroom Physical Activity Intervention Studies (N=9 Studies)* | Total # of Performance Outcomes Across the 9 Intervention Studies | Type of Relationship Observed Between Classroom Physical Activity and Academic Performance | | |
|---|---|---|---|---|
| | | Positive | None | Negative |
| **Cognitive Skills and Attitudes (N=5 Studies)** | **11** | **2** | **9** | **0** |
| Attention/concentration | 2 | 1 | 1 | 0 |
| Visual/spatial skills | 4 | 1 | 3 | 0 |
| Memory | 1 | 0 | 1 | 0 |
| Verbal/conceptual ability | 1 | 0 | 1 | 0 |
| Perceptual/motor ability (coordination) | 2 | 0 | 2 | 0 |
| Mood | 1 | 0 | 1 | 0 |
| **Academic Behavior (N=1 Study)** | **1** | **1** | **0** | **0** |
| Conduct (classroom behavior) | 1 | 1 | 0 | 0 |
| **Academic Achievement (N=6 Studies)** | **8** | **5** | **3** | **0** |
| Achievement test scores (e.g., math, reading, language arts) | 8 | 5 | 3 | 0 |
| **Total** | **20** | **8** | **12** | **0** |

* One qualitative study (Lowden[68]) and one quantitative study (Maeda and Randall[62]) that did not include significance testing were not included in these results. Studies may have measured the relationship between classroom physical activity and academic performance in more than one way (e.g., measured the associations among classroom physical activities and ability, classroom behaviors, and standardized test scores). Individual studies in this section measured between 1 and 11 different outcomes.

16 months and was designed to complement 80 minutes of weekly physical education. Analyses by gender showed similar results.

Collectively, eight of the nine studies reviewed suggest that classroom-based physical activities may have favorable associations with indicators of cognitive functioning, academic behaviors, and/or academic achievement. Furthermore, there was no evidence that allotting classroom time for these activities was negatively associated with academic achievement.

**Strengths and Limitations of Methods.** These studies feature both strengths and important limitations. Eight of the nine studies employed either experimental or quasi-experimental designs, and most used standardized measures of cognitive functioning and academic achievement and standardized protocols for classroom observations. Several studies collected data at multiple follow-up dates. When reported, study populations represented an array of racial and ethnic backgrounds. Limitations reported by study authors include small sample sizes, with all but two studies having fewer than 100 students, and the inability to analyze data by SES, race/ethnicity, or other subgroups. Others noted that classroom observers typically were not blinded to study condition. Some authors also noted concerns about group comparability at baseline and its potential impact on determining an intervention effect.

# Extracurricular Physical Activity Studies

Nineteen studies (reported in 14 articles) examined the relationship between involvement in extracurricular physical activity (such as interscholastic sports or other physical activities outside of the regular school day) and academic performance (see Figure 5, and Tables 5a and 5b). Nine studies focused on involvement in school interscholastic sport teams; the other 10 focused on other school-related extracurricular physical activities. Appendix G includes summary profiles for each of the 14 articles reviewed in this section.

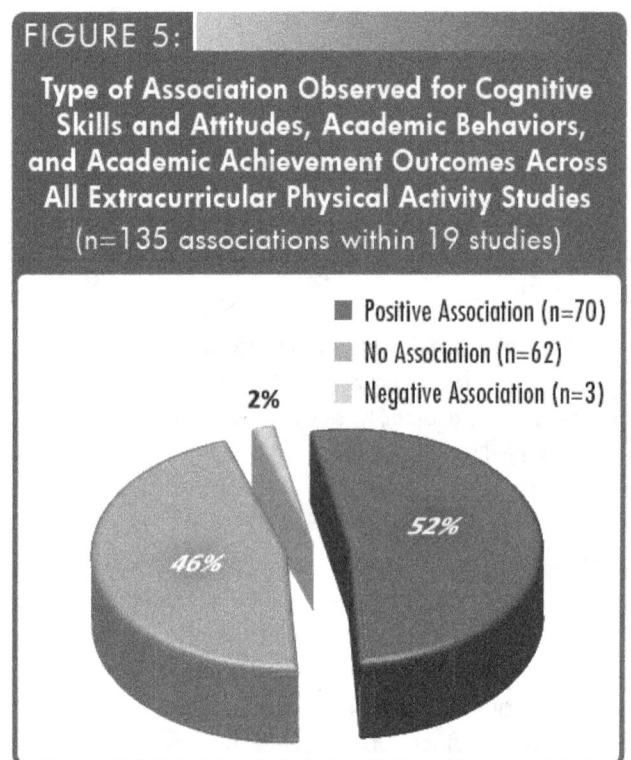

**FIGURE 5:**

**Type of Association Observed for Cognitive Skills and Attitudes, Academic Behaviors, and Academic Achievement Outcomes Across All Extracurricular Physical Activity Studies**
(n=135 associations within 19 studies)

- Positive Association (n=70)
- No Association (n=62)
- Negative Association (n=3)

2%
52%
46%

## Interscholastic School Sports

All nine of the studies assessing the relationship between school sports team participation and academic performance were descriptive in nature and focused on secondary school students.[69-77] Most studies (n=8) were implemented in the United States. Eight of the nine studies examined how students' participation on sports teams was related to test scores, grades, or teacher ratings of academic achievement; two[75,77] measured dropout rates.

## Extracurricular Physical Activity Studies: Highlights

- *Nearly all the associations between extracurricular physical activity and indicators of academic performance were either positive (52%) or neutral (46%).*

- *Grade point average was positively associated with extracurricular physical activity 12 of the 22 times it was measured.*

- *The two different interventions aimed at improving academic performance through extracurricular physical activity had some positive impacts on students' grades and/or verbal and conceptual skills.*

- *Two studies examined the relationship between extracurricular physical activity and dropout rates and found that participation was associated with decreased high school dropout rates.*

Three of the nine studies were cross-sectional, collecting data at one time point; six were longitudinal and involved a secondary analysis of data collected at baseline and 3–5 years later. Two of the nine studies had small samples (85–136); the remaining studies had larger sample sizes (883–14,249).

These studies varied in measurement of academic performance and participation in sports. Some used school records (test scores, GPAs, or dropout rates),[72,74,75,77] and one used a teacher rating of student academic ability[71] for students who participated in interscholastic sports. Others examined the relationship between student report of participation on sports teams (type of team was not specified) and students' self-reported grades.[69,70,73,78]

The studies that explored the relationship between school records of academic achievement and student participation in interscholastic sports found mostly positive and neutral results. For example, one study[74] of eighth-grade students found that participation in interscholastic sports was associated with higher math grades, higher math standardized test scores, and higher overall GPAs; however, another study[72] of 12th-grade students found no relationship between varsity sports participation and grades. Two studies[75,77] examined the impact of sports on high school dropout rates and found that participants were significantly less likely to drop out of school compared with nonparticipants.

Two studies[75,76] found that the relationship between academic achievement and varsity sports participation was inconsistent, showing positive, negative, and no association, depending on the outcome measured and the grade level of the students. Fredricks and Eccles[76] found participation in seventh-grade school sports was associated with a decreased school value in eighth and 11th grades but was associated with increased resiliency in 11th grade. Yin and Moore[75] found that students who reported participation in interscholastic sports in eighth grade showed significantly lower test scores for that year compared with students who did not participate. However, as these same students moved through high school, those differences disappeared, showing no differences in test scores between sport participants and nonparticipants in the 10th or 12th grades. Hawkins and Mulkey's[71] exploration of the relationship between interscholastic sports participation and teacher ratings of students' academic ability showed no relationship between participation and academic ability; however, other measures of academic behavior and cognitive skills and attitudes showed positive relationships or no relationship, varying by gender. As an example, male athletes were more likely to plan to attend college than nonathletes, and both male and female athletes showed greater interest in class than nonathletes.

Three of the four studies that examined the relationship between student report of participation in sports teams and self-report of grades showed positive relationships. Fredricks and Eccles[70] also found a positive relationship between sports participation and students' educational expectations and school completion rates.

Seven of the nine studies examined gender effects[69-72,74,75,76] on academic performance; five of the seven studies found at least one significant difference by gender; however, overall, 68% of the associations by gender showed no relationship. One study[76] also examined results by race and SES. No other subgroup or demographic analyses were reported in the other studies.

## Other School-Related Extracurricular Physical Activity

Ten studies focused on extracurricular physical activities organized through the school but conducted outside the regular school day (e.g., after school). Seven studies examined the effects of an intervention,[2,34] and the other three were descriptive,[79,80,78] with sample sizes ranging from 35 to 4,264. Measures of academic performance included grades, math scores, homework completion, and attendance.

**Intervention Studies.** One intervention article[2] focused on physical activity opportunities after school using six different studies. This article, which focused on studies conducted in the United States, assessed the impact of a life skills program with an emphasis on improving physical fitness on students' self-reported grades, school attendance, and self-concept. The program was taught after school in a sample of middle schools, high schools, and community centers. As part of the program, students completed an individual exercise program as well as instruction about related topics such as self-assessment, goal setting, fitness, and exercise planning. Program impact was evaluated at six sites immediately after the program. Results showed positive associations between program participation and academic performance (grades and attendance) or no significant relationships. The positive findings (for self-concept, school attendance, and self-reported grades) were concentrated in the community site, which had the largest sample size. Across all sites (middle schools, high schools, and community centers), self-concept improved significantly for program participants.

The other intervention study was conducted in the United Kingdom and examined participation in a school-organized, year-long exercise program completed at home and its relationship with cognitive skills and math

## Table 5a: Extracurricular Physical Activity Intervention Studies: Summary of the Outcomes of Cognitive Skills and Attitudes, Academic Behavior, and Academic Achievement

| Variables in Extracurricular Physical Activity Intervention Studies (N=7 Studies)* | Total # of Performance Outcomes Across the 7 Intervention Studies | Type of Relationship Observed Between Extracurricular Physical Activity and Academic Performance | | |
|---|---|---|---|---|
| | | Positive | None | Negative |
| **Cognitive Skills and Attitudes (N=7 Studies)** | **17** | **12** | **5** | **0** |
| Self-esteem/self-concept | 6 | 6 | 0 | 0 |
| Verbal/literacy ability | 8 | 3 | 5 | 0 |
| Working memory | 1 | 1 | 0 | 0 |
| Motor ability (coordination) | 2 | 2 | 0 | 0 |
| **Academic Behavior (N=6 Studies)** | **6** | **1** | **5** | **0** |
| Attendance | 6 | 1 | 5 | 0 |
| **Academic Achievement (N=6 Studies)** | **6** | **1** | **5** | **0** |
| Grade point average | 6 | 1 | 5 | 0 |
| **Total** | **29** | **14** | **15** | **0** |

\* Studies may have measured the relationship between extracurricular physical activity and academic and cognitive performance in more than one way (e.g., measured the association between extracurricular physical activity and grade point average, self-concept, and attendance). Individual studies in this section measured between 3 and 11 different academic measures. Consequently, the number of studies across the three academic performance areas exceeds 2.

outcomes of 7- to 10-year-old children diagnosed with, or at risk of, dyslexia or dyspraxia.[34] This study used a quasi-experimental design with immediate and long-term (3-year) follow-up. Little detail was provided on how the physical activity intervention was developed or implemented. Children showed improved verbal and cognitive skills following the individualized physical activity intervention, although there were no math improvements.[34]

**Nonintervention Studies.** The three nonintervention studies, all conducted with secondary students in the United States, examined associations between participation in after-school physical activity and academic performance using existing data sets (one cross-sectional and two longitudinal). Two studies[78,79] explored the association between student reports of participation in extracurricular activities and student self-reported grades, including involvement in a combination of sports and nonsport activities. Those studies found consistently positive associations between extracurricular activity participation and self-reported grades as well

as positive academic attitudes and higher academic aspirations. Harrison and Narayan[80] examined the impact of participation in after-school activities (including participating 1–2 hours per week or more in school sports) on homework completion and class attendance. The study showed that physical activity participation was positively related to homework completion and class attendance.

**Strengths and Limitations of Methods.** These studies featured a number of strengths. Most had relatively large sample sizes. Most (n=16) of the studies focused on measures of academic achievement, such as standardized test scores or grades (record data or self-reported data). In addition, of the studies that examined sports participation compared with nonparticipation, more than half (n=6) specified the level of competitiveness of team participation; nonetheless, these studies did not compare outcomes by varying levels of sports competitiveness. More than three-fourths of the studies were longitudinal in nature (n=15), allowing for an exploration of causality; the cross-sectional nature of the remaining studies (n=4) limited the ability to establish the temporal relationship between the variables. Relatively few studies examined data by race/ethnicity, and only two explored physical activity interventions. Reports were unclear whether sport participation required a minimal level of academic achievement, a requirement that could bias the samples.

Several authors also acknowledged limitations such as the need to include measures of social influence (e.g., parental support) in future research, the need to look more closely at how level of participation or competitiveness in sport might affect academic achievement, and the fact that some of the associations found were relatively weak.

## Table 5b: Extracurricular Physical Activity Nonintervention Studies: Summary of the Outcomes of Cognitive Skills and Attitudes, Academic Behavior, and Academic Achievement

| Variables in Extracurricular Physical Activity Intervention Studies (N=12 Studies)* | Total # of Performance Outcomes Across the 12 Intervention Studies | Type of Relationship Observed Between Extracurricular Physical Activity and Academic Performance | | |
| --- | --- | --- | --- | --- |
| | | Positive | None | Negative |
| **Cognitive Skills and Attitudes (N=7 Studies)** | **48** | **28** | **18** | **2** |
| Self-esteem/self-efficacy/self-concept | 19 | 5 | 4 | 0 |
| Academic self-concept/competence | 3 | 2 | 1 | 0 |
| Locus of control | 5 | 4 | 1 | 0 |
| Educational aspirations/potential | 4 | 4 | 0 | 0 |
| Interest in class | 4 | 3 | 1 | 0 |
| Mood | 8 | 1 | 7 | 0 |
| Positive academic attitudes | 3 | 3 | 0 | 0 |
| School value | 4 | 0 | 2 | 2 |
| School attachment | 4 | 4 | 0 | 0 |
| Resiliency | 4 | 2 | 2 | 0 |
| **Academic Behavior (N=3 Studies)** | **34** | **15** | **19** | **0** |
| Conduct (discipline) | 4 | 0 | 4 | 0 |
| Enrollment in academic track/science class | 4 | 2 | 2 | 0 |
| School completion | 1 | 1 | 0 | 0 |
| Attendance | 6 | 2 | 4 | 0 |
| Prepared for class | 4 | 0 | 4 | 0 |
| Homework completion | 2 | 2 | 0 | 0 |
| Attend college | 4 | 2 | 2 | 0 |
| Dropout rates/graduation | 9 | 6 | 3 | 0 |
| **Academic Achievement (N=10 Studies)** | **24** | **13** | **10** | **1** |
| Achievement test scores (e.g., math, reading, language arts) | 4 | 1 | 2 | 1 |
| Grade point average/grades | 16 | 11 | 5 | 0 |
| Academic ability | 4 | 1 | 3 | 0 |
| **Total** | **106** | **56** | **47** | **3** |

\* Studies may have measured the relationship between extracurricular physical activity and academic performance in more than one way (e.g., measured the association between participation in sports and test scores, attendance, and perceived academic potential). Individual studies in this section measured between 1 and 32 different academic measures. Consequently, the number of studies across the three academic performance areas exceeds 14.

# SUMMARY

This report identified peer-reviewed studies and published reports addressing the association between physical activity, including physical education, and indicators of academic performance, including those related to cognitive skills and attitudes, academic behaviors, and academic achievement.

## Overall Findings

### Overall, what do the results of these studies say about the relationship between physical activity and academics, and what does it mean for schools?

- Collectively, the results suggest that physical activity is either positively related to academic performance (50.5% of the associations summarized) or that there is not a demonstrated relationship between physical activity and academic performance (48% of the associations summarized). In addition, increasing time during the school day for physical activity does not appear to take away from academic performance. This pattern of having positive relationships or no relationships, along with the lack of negative relationships, was consistent throughout the results, despite the heterogeneous nature of the included studies, and is consistent with other published reviews.[15,81]

- School boards, school administrators, and principals can feel confident that maintaining or increasing time dedicated for physical activity during the school day will not have a negative impact on academic performance, and it may positively impact students' academic performance.

### What kinds of academic outcomes were positively related to physical activity?

- Studies looked at a broad range of outcomes. Researchers reported that participating in physical activity was positively related to outcomes including academic achievement, academic behaviors, and indicators of cognitive skills and attitudes, such as concentration, memory, self-esteem, and verbal skills.

### Which outcomes were most positive?

- Positive associations were found across measures of academic achievement, academic behavior, and cognitive skills and attitudes, but there are some interesting patterns for different outcomes within these categories. Seven articles describing intervention studies (three school-based physical education, two recess, one classroom-based physical activity, and one extracurricular activity) evaluated the relationship between physical activity and academic behaviors, such as classroom conduct.[2,41,42,50,56,57,63] The majority of these articles (86%) found at least one positive association with academic behavior outcomes. Given these findings, physical activity interventions may offer one approach to improving academic behaviors (e.g., classroom conduct) in some youth.

### Does physical activity have any negative relationship with grades or test scores?

- Very few of the findings in the studies reviewed were negative (only 4 associations of 251 examined), a percentage small enough to reasonably be expected by chance. This pattern of results is consistent with other reports[15,16] that suggest that adding physical activity to the school day does not detract from academic performance. The evidence suggests that superintendents and principals can devote school time to physical activity without concern that it will lower student test scores.

### Why are some of the study results positive whereas others show no relationship?

- There are a number of possible explanations. Some of the studies had relatively small samples, which can make it more difficult to find statistically significant results. Other studies measured a very broad range of student attitudes and behaviors to try to understand which factors may be related and *which may not*. Other issues, such as the questionnaires used in the studies, may account for some of the differences. Finally, differences that may not have been discussed in the studies—such as the intensity or duration of the physical activity, the context in which the physical activity took place, individual student differences (e.g., in motivation), and levels and quality of implementation for intervention studies—may help explain the different results among the studies.

# Findings for Physical Activity by Context

## Is school-based physical education related to academic performance?

- The study results suggest that school-based physical education either leads to a positive result or is associated with no change in academic performance. Overall, 11 of 14 studies found one or more positive associations between physical education and indicators of cognitive skills and attitudes, academic behavior, and/or academic achievement. Nearly half the associations (49.5%) between physical education and academic performance were positive; nearly all remaining associations in this context area showed no relationship.

- The studies also suggest that increased time spent in physical education is not likely to detract from academic performance even when less time is devoted to subjects other than physical education. Across the nine studies that examined the relationship between time spent in physical education and academic performance, 16 outcomes were positive and 31 showed no association. No negative associations were found.

## Is recess related to academic performance?

- Yes, for some outcomes. Eight studies meeting the criteria of this review looked at the impact of physical activity during recess on academic performance. Of all outcomes measured in this context area, 59% were positive. In addition, all eight studies found one or more positive findings suggesting that recess was associated with improvements in attention, concentration, and/or on-task classroom behavior. None of the studies looked directly at the association between recess and measures of academic achievement (e.g., test scores or grades).

- None of the studies reported negative relationships, which indicates that recess does not appear to detract from students' focus in the classroom.

## Are physical activity breaks during class related to academic performance?

- Yes, for some outcomes. Nearly all studies (eight of nine) in this category found that offering physical activity breaks during standard classroom instruction may have favorable associations with some indicators of cognitive functioning (e.g., attention/concentration); academic behaviors (e.g., classroom conduct); and/or academic achievement (e.g., test scores). Of the individual outcomes studied, 40% of associations between physical activity breaks and academic performance were positive and 60% showed no relationship.

- None of the studies found negative associations. Classroom physical activity breaks do not appear to have a negative relationship with academic performance. Indeed, classroom teachers can include physical activity breaks as one strategy to promote academic-related benefits for students. Furthermore, incorporating brief physical activity breaks into the classroom might contribute to students' overall levels of physical activity and health.[82]

## Is participation in extracurricular physical activities at school related to academic performance?

- Yes, for some outcomes. More than half of the associations examined in these studies were positive (52% overall), and almost none were negative (2%). Of note, GPA was positively associated with extracurricular physical activity 12 of the 22 times it was measured. Two studies also examined the association between extracurricular activities and dropout rates and found that participation was linked to decreased high school dropout rates.

# Findings by Gender, Other Demographic Characteristics, and Research Design

## Do the results vary by gender?

- Relatively few studies examined differences in associations by gender, and there were no distinct patterns. Of studies that did examine data by gender, a few found differences, but most did not. For example, eight of the studies on school-based physical education examined data by gender. Six found no differences by gender; one found effects favoring boys (higher-level motor skills were associated with greater increases in reading and math scores among boys than girls); and one found effects favoring girls (greater time spent in physical education was related to higher reading and math scores for girls but not for boys).

## How do the studies and results differ by grade level?

- Studies of recess and classroom-based physical activity tended to be from elementary school settings, and studies of extracurricular physical activity tended to be from secondary school settings.
- Overall, the pattern of results appeared slightly more positive in the secondary school setting. Of the associations examined among elementary youth only, 43% were positive, 56% were neutral, and 1% were negative. At the secondary level, 55% of the associations examined were positive, 43% were neutral, and 2% were negative.

## Do the results vary by race/ethnicity?

- Very few studies examined the relationships between physical activity and academic performance by race or ethnicity, so it is difficult to make conclusions at this time. Of the seven studies that explored race/ethnicity, most focused on how race/ethnicity affected participation in physical activity rather than on how it influenced the association between physical activity and academic achievement. One study examining classroom-based physical activity breaks by race found

no differences in academic performance between Asian and Caucasian students.[65] A study of an 8-week movement intervention found that language spoken (Afrikaans, English, and Other), used as a proxy indicator for race/ethnicity, may have explained some differences in children's spatial aptitude.[66]

## Do the results vary by research design?

- Not much variation in results by research design was noted. Although many factors influence a study's quality, experimental or quasi-experimental research designs are generally regarded as more rigorous. The pattern of associations in studies with either of these types of design had very similar results. In the 29 studies using experimental or quasi-experimental designs, 50% (55 of 109) of associations were positive, and 49% (53 of 109) were not significant. Less than 1% (1 of 109) of the associations were negative.

# Strengths and Limitations of Review

## What are the strengths of this review?

- This review has a number of strengths. It covers 23 years of research; it involved a systematic process for locating, reviewing, and coding the studies; articles were obtained using an extensive array of search terms and international databases; articles were reviewed by multiple trained coders; and the articles cover a broad array of contexts in which youth participate in school-based physical activities. Furthermore, a majority (64%) of studies included in the review were intervention studies, and a majority (76%) were longitudinal.

## What are the limitations of this review?

- This review summarizes all studies that met the established review criteria, regardless of the study characteristics. The studies were not ranked, weighted, or grouped according to their strengths and limitations; as a result, findings from studies with more rigorous research designs and larger sample sizes were given no more influence than findings from studies with weaker designs and smaller sample sizes. Instead, results were based on counts of statistical findings, and this, in essence, had the effect of allowing individual studies containing multiple comparisons to have a greater influence on the findings as a whole. The number of statistical findings in any given study ranged from 1 to 32; given those differences, it becomes clear that a single study with 32 comparisons would have influenced the overall results more than a study that included only 1 comparison.

In addition, the breadth of the review, while revealing a variety of study designs, measures, and populations, often made comparisons and summaries difficult. For example, similar constructs were often defined and/or measured differently across studies. Even something as seemingly consistent as standardized test scores can vary from state to state. Therefore, these inconsistencies limit the ability of this or any review to draw specific conclusions across all studies.

For the same reason, it was not appropriate to make broad statements about effect sizes. Although the studies in this review include examples of moderate and large effect sizes,[47,51,63] there were not enough studies analyzing the same variables in any given category to make summary statements about the magnitude of associations between physical activity and academic performance variables. As a result, conclusions do not summarize magnitudes of effect sizes and are intentionally broad.

# Implications for Future Research or Evaluation

### What other research or evaluation needs to be done to further the field in this area?

- Within the contexts reviewed, there were relatively few studies of the impact of recess and classroom physical activity on academic achievement. None of the reviewed studies examined the relationship of sports and academic achievement within the primary grades or the relationship of physically active breaks/recess and academic achievement within the secondary grades. Few studies conducted subgroup analyses beyond gender comparisons.

- Less than half of the studies described effect sizes or magnitudes of the associations observed. Reporting of effect sizes can guide researchers and practitioners towards interventions most likely to impact outcomes of interest.

- Although nearly all of the reviewed studies described a practical framework for the research, few of the studies articulated a theoretical basis for the work or explicitly described how the findings informed theory development. Theoretical specificity may enable researchers to more easily identify relevant bodies of work from other disciplines, consider new relationships and mechanisms of action, align and strengthen intervention design and measurement, and ultimately progress the field more effectively and efficiently.

- Improved understanding of the specific cognitive and behavioral impacts of particular physical activities could inform intervention developers and improve the match between interventions, populations, and educational goals. For example, compared with measures of cognitive skills and attitudes, academic behaviors such as on-task classroom behavior or following instructions were less likely to be examined as proximal outcomes of physical activity or potential mediators of academic achievement.

- Future research should further examine the relationship between school-based physical activity and academic performance in subpopulations of students (e.g., based on gender, race/ethnicity, or SES). Results from this type of research could help physical education teachers and physical activity coordinators apply findings of programs and interventions to meet the needs of particular groups of students.

- Future research should be developed in consultation with educators (e.g., school administrators and staff) and informed by research across disciplines, such as neurobiology, cognitive science, social psychology, and kinesiology. For instance, few studies placed the work within a neurobiology model to better understand the role of brain physiology, within an ecological framework to account for contextual variables, or within a developmental perspective to examine developmental differences in relationships between physical activity and academic achievement.

- Future research and evaluation would benefit from identifying uniform ways to measure key outcomes, including both physical activity and academic performance outcomes. Similarly, future studies would benefit from larger sample sizes and stronger research designs that include longitudinal follow-up, as appropriate. Adequate follow-up of interventions has been more limited in physical education compared with other contexts.

## Implications for Schools

### What are the policy and practice implications from this review?

- Schools should continue to offer or increase opportunities for physical activity. There is evidence that physical activity may help improve academic performance (including grades and standardized test scores) in some situations. Increasing or maintaining time dedicated to physical education does not adversely impact academic performance.

- The studies in this review also suggest that physical activity can impact cognitive skills and attitudes, important components of improved academic performance. This includes enhanced concentration and attention as well as improved classroom behavior.

- Taking all of the evidence into account, schools should strive to meet the National Association for Sport and Physical Education's recommendation of daily physical education and offer students a balanced academic program that includes opportunities for a variety of daily physical activities.

### What are the current recommendations for students' physical activity?

- Recent recommendations indicate that 6- to 17-year-olds should be participating in at least 60 minutes of physical activity daily,[83] and schools can and should provide opportunities for physical activity to help students meet this recommendation. In fact, the Institute of Medicine's *Preventing Childhood Obesity: Health in the Balance* report recommended that schools provide a significant portion of students' daily physical activity.[84]

- To enable students to meet these recommended levels of physical activity, the National Association for Sport and Physical Education recommends that all pre-K through grade 12 schools implement a comprehensive school physical activity program, which includes quality physical education; physical activity before, during, and after school, including recess and other physical activity breaks; extracurricular, noncompetitive physical activity clubs; interscholastic sports; and walk- and bike-to-school initiatives.[35]

### How can schools promote physical activity at school?

- Physical activity can be included in the school environment in a number of ways without detracting from academic performance. Studies highlight potential benefits of physical activity in physical education classes, during recess, in regular classrooms, and through extracurricular sports and other physical activity opportunities.

  - *School-based physical education:* To maximize the potential benefits of student participation in physical education class, schools and physical education teachers can consider increasing the amount of time students spend in physical education class or adding components to increase the quality of physical education class. Studies reviewed here showed that programs were able to increase physical education time by increasing the number of days per week or the length of class time, adding trained physical education instructors, supplementing programs with community resources, and using outside facilities (e.g., swimming pools). In addition, the studies reviewed here explored several different strategies for enhancing the quality of physical education class, requiring varying levels of resources. These range from implementing a standards- and research-based physical education curriculum to adding specific components to physical education.

  - *Recess:* Studies reviewed here used structured or unstructured play during recess as a means to provide students with time for movement and play during the school day. School boards, superintendents, principals, and teachers can feel confident that providing recess to students on a regular basis may benefit academic behaviors (e.g., attention), facilitate social development,[85] and contribute to overall physical activity[86] and its associated health benefits.

- *Classroom-based physical activity:* Movement activities and physical activity breaks are simple ways for classroom teachers to enhance student physical activity and possibly academic performance. Most interventions described in this review used short breaks (5–20 minutes) that required little or no teacher preparation, special equipment, or resources. As an example, interventions such as speed (cup) stacking could be a center or activity station. Simple movement-based learning techniques (e.g., walking around the perimeter of the classroom while learning vocabulary or using music and rhythmic movement to enhance memory tasks) could be incorporated into large group lessons. Short exercise breaks (e.g., 5 minutes of walking or 10 minutes of prescribed exercise) could be introduced into the classroom routine prior to teaching subjects that require intense student concentration.

- *Extracurricular physical activities:* The evidence in this review suggests that superintendents, principals, and athletic directors can develop or continue school-based sports programs (e.g., intramurals or physical activity clubs and interscholastic sports programs), without concern that participation in such activities would have negative associations with academic performance. Increasing or maintaining time dedicated to physical activity does not adversely impact academic performance. Indeed, studies suggest there may be a range of possible benefits for some students, including developing a stronger sense of self, fostering educational aspirations, maintaining interest in class, encouraging homework completion, and reducing dropout rates. School administrators and teachers can also encourage after-school organizations, clubs, student groups, and parent groups to incorporate physical activities into their programs and events (e.g., fundraisers, special activities).

• Collectively, the findings from this review support the National Association for Sport and Physical Education's recommendations for a comprehensive school physical activity program.[35] The results also suggest that physical education and physical activity may help advance academic performance for many students and should not hinder academic progress.

# REFERENCES

1. Physical Activity Guidelines Advisory Committee. *Physical Activity Guidelines Advisory Committee Report, 2008.* Washington, DC: U.S. Department of Health and Human Services; 2008.

2. Collingwood TR, Sunderlin J, Reynolds R, Kohl HW 3rd. Physical training as a substance abuse prevention intervention for youth. *Journal of Drug Education* 2000;30(4):435–451.

3. Strong WB, Malina RM, Blimkie CJR, et al. Evidence based physical activity for school-age youth. *Journal of Pediatrics* 2005;146(6):732–737.

4. National Center for Education Statistics. *Digest of Education Statistics: 2008.* Washington, DC: National Center for Education Statistics; 2009.

5. Wilkins JLM, Graham G, Parker S, Westfall S, Fraser RG, Tembo M. Time in the arts and physical education and school achievement. *Journal of Curriculum Studies* 2003;35(6): 721–734.

6. Centers for Disease Control and Prevention. Youth risk behavior surveillance—United States, 2007. *MMWR* 2008;57(SS-4):1–131.

7. Lee SM, Burgeson CR, Fulton JE, Spain CG. Physical education and physical activity: results from the School Health Policies and Programs Study 2006. *Journal of School Health* 2007;77(8):435–463.

8. Coatsworth JD, Conroy DE. Youth sport as a component of organized afterschool programs. *New Directions for Youth Development* 2007(115):57–74.

9. Hofferth S, Curtin S. Leisure time activities in middle childhood. In: Moore KA, Lippman LH, eds. *What Do Children Need to Flourish?* New York: Springer;2005:95–110.

10. Castelli DM, Hillman CH, Buck SM, Erwin HE. Physical fitness and academic achievement in third- and fifth-grade students. *Journal of Sport and Exercise Psychology* 2007;29(2):239–252.

11. Trudeau F, Shephard RJ. Relationships of physical activity to brain health and the academic performance of schoolchildren. *American Journal of Lifestyle Medicine* 2010;4(2):138–150.

12. Sibley BA, Etnier JL. The relationship between physical activity and cognition in children: a meta-analysis. *Pediatric Exercise Science* 2003;15(3):243–256.

13. Taras H. Physical activity and student performance at school. *Journal of School Health* 2005;75(6):214–218.

14. Tomporowski PD, Davis CL, Miller PH, Naglieri JA. Exercise and children's intelligence, cognition, and academic achievement. *Educational Psychology Review* 2008;20(2):111–131.

15. Trost S. *Active Education: Physical Education, Physical Activity and Academic Performance.* San Diego, CA: Active Living Research; 2007.

16. Trudeau F, Shephard RJ. Physical education, school physical activity, school sports and academic performance. *International Journal of Behavioral Nutrition and Physical Activity;*2008:5(10).

17. Hillman CH, Castelli DM, Buck SM. Aerobic fitness and neurocognitive function in healthy preadolescent children. *Medicine and Science in Sports and Exercise* 2005;37(11):1967–1974.

18. Rosenbaum DA, Carlson RA, Gilmore RO. Acquisition of intellectual and perceptual-motor skills. *Annual Review of Psychology* 2001;52:453–470.

19. Smith LB, Thelen E, Titzer R, McLin D. Knowing in the context of acting: the task dynamics of the A-not-B error. *Psychological Review* 1999;106(2):235–260.

20. Hillman CH, Erickson KI, Kramer AF. Be smart, exercise your heart: exercise effects on brain and cognition. *Nature Reviews Neuroscience* 2008;9(1):58–65.

21. California Department of Education. *California Physical Fitness Test: A Study of the Relationship between Physical Fitness and Academic Achievement in California Using 2004 Test Results.* Sacramento, CA: California Department of Education; 2005.

22. Dwyer T, Sallis JF, Blizzard L, Lazarus R, Dean K. Relation of academic performance to physical activity and fitness in children. *Pediatric Exercise Science* 2001;13(3):225–237.

23. Grissom JB. Physical fitness and academic achievement. *Journal of Exercise Physiology Online;*2005:11–25.

24. Kim H-YP, Frongillo EA, Han S-S, et al. Academic performance of Korean children is associated with dietary behaviours and physical status. *Asia Pacific Journal of Clinical Nutrition* 2003;12(2):186–192.
25. Martin LT, Chalmers GR. The relationship between academic achievement and physical fitness. *Physical Educator* 2007;64(4):214–221.
26. Sollerhed AC, Ejlertsson G. Low physical capacity among adolescents in practical education. *Scandinavian Journal of Medicine and Science in Sports* 1999;9(5):249–256.
27. Themane MJ, Koppes LLJ, Kemper HCG, Monyeki KD, Twisk JWR. The relationship between physical activity, fitness and educational achievement of rural South African children. *Journal of Physical Education and Recreation* 2006;12(1):48–54.
28. Buck SM, Hillman CH, Castelli DM. The relation of aerobic fitness to Stroop task performance in preadolescent children. *Medicine and Science in Sports and Exercise* 2007;40(1):166–172.
29. Knight D, Rizzuto T. Relations for children in grades 2, 3, and 4 between balance skills and academic achievement. *Perceptual and Motor Skills* 1993;76(3 Pt 2):1296–1298.
30. Nourbakhsh P. Perceptual-motor abilities and their relationships with academic performance of fifth grade pupils in comparison with Oseretsky scale. *Kinesiology* 2006;38(1):40–48.
31. Son S-H, Meisels SJ. The relationship of young children's motor skills to later reading and math achievement. *Merrill Palmer Quarterly* 2006;52(4):755–778.
32. Boykin AW, Allen BA. Rhythmic-movement facilitation of learning in working-class Afro-American children. *Journal of Genetic Psychology* 1988;149(3):335–347.
33. Oja L, Jürimäe T. Physical activity, motor ability, and school readiness of 6-yr.-old children. *Perceptual and Motor Skills* 2002;95(2):407–415.
34. Reynolds D, Nicolson RI. Follow-up of an exercise-based treatment for children with reading difficulties. *Dyslexia* 2007;13(2):78–96.
35. National Association for Sport and Physical Education. *Comprehensive School Physical Activity Programs.* Reston, VA: National Association for Sport and Physical Education; 2008.
36. Centers for Disease Control and Prevention. *School Connectedness: Strategies for Increasing Protective Factors among Youth.* Atlanta, GA: Centers for Disease Control and Prevention; 2009.
37. Pellegrini AD, Huberty PD, Jones I. The effects of recess timing on children's playground and classroom behaviors. *American Educational Research Journal* 1995;32(4):845–864.
38. Kirby DB. *Emerging Answers 2007: Research Findings on Programs to Reduce Teen Pregnancy and Sexually Transmitted Diseases.* Washington, DC: National Campaign to Prevent Teen and Unwanted Pregnancy; 2007.
39. Stone EJ, McKenzie TL, Welk GJ, Booth ML. Effects of physical activity interventions in youth. Review and synthesis. *American Journal of Preventive Medicine* 1998;15(4):298–315.
40. Welk GJ, Corbin CB, Dale D. Measurement issues in the assessment of physical activity in children. *Research Quarterly for Exercise and Sport* 2000;71(2 Suppl):S59–S73.
41. Bluechardt MH, Wiener J, Shephard RJ. Exercise programmes in the treatment of children with learning disabilities. *Sports Medicine* 1995;19(1):55–72.
42. Dwyer T, Blizzard L, Dean K. Physical activity and performance in children. *Nutrition Reviews* 1996;54 (4 Pt 2):S27–S31.
43. Ericsson I. Motor skills, attention and academic achievements: an intervention study in school years 1-3. *British Educational Research Journal* 2008;34(3):301–313.
44. McNaughten D, Gabbard C. Physical exertion and immediate mental performance of sixth-grade children. *Perceptual and Motor Skills* 1993;77(3 Pt 2):1155–1159.
45. Pollatschek JL, O'Hagan FJ. An investigation of the psycho-physical influences of a quality daily physical education programme. *Health Education Research* 1989;4(3):341–350.
46. Raviv S, Low M. Influence of physical activity on concentration among junior high-school students. *Perceptual and Motor Skills* 1990;70(1):67–74.

47. Milosis D, Papaioannou AG. Interdisciplinary teaching, multiple goals and self-concept. In: Liukkonen J, Vanden Auweele Y, Vereijken B, Alfermann D, Theodorakis Y, eds. *Psychology for Physical Educators: Student in Focus.* 2nd ed. Champaign, IL: Human Kinetics;2007:175–198.

48. Sallis JF, McKenzie TL, Kolody B, Lewis M, Marshall S, Rosengard P. Effects of health-related physical education on academic achievement: Project SPARK. *Research Quarterly for Exercise and Sport* 1999;70(2):127–134.

49. Budde H, Voelcker-Rehage C, Pietraßyk-Kendziorra S, Ribeiro P, Tidow G. Acute coordinative exercise improves attentional performance in adolescents. *Neuroscience Letters* 2008;441(2):219–223.

50. Tuckman BW, Hinkle JS. An experimental study of the physical and psychological effects of aerobic exercise on schoolchildren. *Health Psychology* 1986;5(3):197–207.

51. Tremarche PV, Robinson EM, Graham LB. Physical education and its effect on elementary testing results. *Physical Educator* 2007;64(2):58–64.

52. Carlson SA, Fulton JE, Lee SM, et al. Physical education and academic achievement in elementary school: data from the Early Childhood Longitudinal Study. *American Journal of Public Health* 2008;98(4):721–727.

53. Dexter T. Relationships between sport knowledge, sport performance and academic ability: empirical evidence from GCSE Physical Education. *Journal of Sports Sciences* 1999;17(4):283–295.

54. Dollman J, Boshoff K, Dodd G. The relationship between curriculum time for physical education and literacy and numeracy standards in South Australian primary schools. *European Physical Education Review* 2006;12(2):151–163.

55. Caterino MC, Polak ED. Effects of two types of activity on the performance of second-, third-, and fourth-grade students on a test of concentration. *Perceptual and Motor Skills* 1999;89(1):245–248.

56. Jarrett OS, Maxwell DM, Dickerson C, Hoge P, Davies G, Yetley A. Impact of recess on classroom behavior: Group effects and individual differences. *Journal of Educational Research* 1998;92(2):121–126.

57. Pellegrini AD, Davis PD. Relations between children's playground and classroom behaviour. *British Journal of Educational Psychology* 1993;63(1):88–95.

58. Barros RM, Silver EJ, Stein RE. School recess and group classroom behavior. *Pediatrics* 2009;123(2): 431–436.

59. Pellegrini AD, Kato K, Blatchford P, Baines E. A short-term longitudinal study of children's playground games across the first year of school: implications for social competence and adjustment to school. *American Educational Research Journal* 2002;39(4):991–1015.

60. Norlander T, Moas L, Archer T. Noise and stress in primary and secondary school children: noise reduction and increased concentration ability through a short but regular exercise and relaxation program. *School Effectiveness and School Improvement* 2005;16(1):91–99.

61. Della Valle J, Dunn R, Geisert G, Sinatra R, Zenhausern R. The effects of matching and mismatching students mobility preferences on recognition and memory tasks. *Journal of Educational Research* 1986;79(5):267–272.

62. Maeda JK, Randall LM. Can academic success come from five minutes of physical activity? *Brock Education* 2003;13(1):14–22.

63. Mahar MT, Murphy SK, Rowe DA, Golden J, Shields AT, Raedeke TD. Effects of a classroom-based program on physical activity and on-task behavior. *Medicine and Science in Sports and Exercise* 2006;38(12):2086–2094.

64. Molloy GN. Chemicals, exercise and hyperactivity: a short report. *International Journal of Disability, Development and Education* 1989;36(1):57–61.

65. Ahamed Y, MacDonald H, Reed K, Naylor P-J, Liu-Ambrose T, McKay H. School-based physical activity does not compromise children's academic performance. *Medicine and Science in Sports and Exercise* 2007;39(2):371–376.

66. Fredericks CR, Kokot SJ, Krog S. Using a developmental movement programme to enhance academic skills in grade 1 learners. *South African Journal of Research in Sport, Physical Education and Recreation* 2006;28(1):29–42.

67. Uhrich TA, Swalm RL. A pilot study of a possible effect from a motor task on reading performance. *Perceptual and Motor Skills* 2007;104(3 Pt 1):1035–1041.

68. Lowden K, Powney J, Davidson J, James C. *The Class Moves! Pilot in Scotland and Wales: An Evaluation.* Edinburgh, Scotland: Scottish Council for Research in Education; 2001.

69. Crosnoe R. Academic and health-related trajectories in adolescence: the intersection of gender and athletics. *Journal of Health and Social Behavior* 2002;43(3):317–335.

70. Fredricks JA, Eccles JS. Is extracurricular participation associated with beneficial outcomes? Concurrent and longitudinal relations. *Developmental Psychology* 2006;42(4):698–713.

71. Hawkins R, Mulkey LM. Athletic investment and academic resilience in a national sample of African American females and males in the middle grades. *Education and Urban Society* 2005;38(1):62–88.

72. Schumaker JF, Small L, Wood J. Self-concept, academic achievement, and athletic participation. *Perceptual and Motor Skills* 1986;62(2):387–390.

73. Spence JC, Poon P. Results from the Alberta Schools' Athletic Association Survey. *Research Update* 1997;5(1).

74. Stephens LJ, Schaben LA. The effect of interscholastic sports participation on academic achievement of middle level school students. *NAASP Bulletin* 2002;86(630):34–41.

75. Yin Z, Moore JB. Re-examining the role of interscholastic sport participation in education. *Psychological Reports* 2004;94(3 Pt 2):1447–1454.

76. Fredricks J, Eccles J. Participation in extracurricular activities in the middle school years: Are there developmental benefits for African American and European American youth? *Journal of Youth and Adolescence* 2008;37(9):1029–1043.

77. McNeal RB, Jr. Extracurricular activities and high school dropouts. *Sociology of Education* 1995;68(1):62–81.

78. Darling N. Participation in extracurricular activities and adolescent adjustment: cross-sectional and longitudinal findings. *Journal of Youth and Adolescence* 2005;34(5):493–505.

79. Darling N, Caldwell LL, Smith R. Participation in school-based extracurricular activities and adolescent adjustment. *Journal of Leisure Research* 2005;37(1):51–76.

80. Harrison PA, Narayan G. Differences in behavior, psychological factors, and environmental factors associated with participation in school sports and other activities in adolescence. *Journal of School Health* 2003;73(3):113–120.

81. Shephard RJ. Curricular physical activity and academic performance. *Pediatric Exercise Science* 1997;9(2):113–126.

82. Stewart JA, Dennison DA, Kohl HW, Doyle AJ. Exercise level and energy expenditure in the TAKE 10! in-class physical activity program. *Journal of School Health* 2004;74(10):397–400.

83. U.S. Department of Health and Human Services. *2008 Physical Activity Guidelines for Americans.* Washington, DC: U.S. Department of Health and Human Services; 2008.

84. Koplan, JP, Liverman, CT, Kraak, VA, editors, Committee on Prevention of Obesity in Children and Youth, National Institute of Medicine. *Preventing Childhood Obesity: Health in the Balance.* Washington, DC: National Academy of Sciences Press; 2005.

85. National Association for Sport and Physical Education. *Recess for elementary school students* [Position paper]. Reston, VA: National Association for Sport and Physical Education; 2006.

86. Ridgers ND, Stratton G, Fairclough SJ. Physical activity levels of children during school playtime. *Sports Medicine (Auckland, NZ)* 2006;36(4):359–371.

87. Vogt WP. *Dictionary of Statistics and Methodology.* Thousand Oaks, CA: Sage Publications; 1999.

88. Bailey KD. *Methods of Social Research.* 4th ed. New York: The Free Press; 1994.

89. Schutt RK. *Investigating the Social World: The Process and Practice of Research.* Thousand Oaks, CA: Pine Forge Press; 1999.

90. Grembowski D. *The Practice of Health Program Evaluation.* Thousand Oaks, CA: Sage Publications; 2001.

91. Trochim WMK. *Experimental Design.* 2006. Available at http://www.socialresearchmethods.net/kb/desexper.php.

92. Centers for Disease Control and Prevention. *HIV Prevention Community Planning Guide.* Atlanta, GA: Centers for Disease Control and Prevention; 2003.

93. Trochim WMK. *Quasi-experimental Design.* 2006. Available at http://www.socialresearchmethods.net/kb/quasiexp.php.

# Appendix A: Database Search Terms

# SEARCH TERMS

## Physical Activity

- Physical activity
- Exercise
- Physical education
- Fitness
- Sport
- Sport participation (searched in Cumulative Index to Nursing and Allied Health Literature [CINAHL®] and SportDiscus™ only)
- Energy expenditure (searched in CINAHL® and SportDiscus™ only)

## Academic-Related

- Academic achievement
- Academic problems
- Educational status (MeSH)
- Education measurement (MeSH)
- Graduation rates
- Academic grades
- Grade point average (GPA)
- Standardized test scores
- Grade retention
- Years of school completed
- Time on task
- Attentiveness
- Concentration (searched in CINAHL® and SportDiscus™ only)
- Attendance
- Tardiness
- Discipline
- Memory
- Reading achievement

- Reading performance
- Mathematics achievement
- Mathematics performance
- Science achievement
- Science performance
- Educational indicators
- Achievement scores
- Educational testing
- Educational assessment
- Dropout
- School refusal
- Student motivation
- Student engagement
- Student learning
- Information retrieval (searched in CINAHL® and SportDiscus™ only)
- Cognitive performance
- Student assessment
- Brain development
- School connectedness

## Databases For Searching

- PubMed
- SportDiscus™
- CINAHL®
- Expanded Academic Index ASAP
- PsycNET®
- Sociological Abstracts
- ERIC
- ScienceDirect®
- Google Scholar

# Appendix B: Coding Sheet

| | |
|---|---|
| Topic: | |
| Title of Article: | |
| Date of Article (month/year): | |
| Citation: <br> Journal: | |
| Authors: | |
| Volume/edition/pages: | |

**1. Purpose of study as stated by author**

**2. Research questions/hypotheses as stated by author**

**3. Study Design (check all that apply)**

| Study Type | | Data Type | |
|---|---|---|---|
| | Quasi-experimental | | Quantitative |
| | Experimental | | Qualitative |
| | Case study | | |
| **Cohort Design** | | **Follow-up Design** | |
| | Cross-sectional | | Immediate post |
| | Prospective | | Delayed post |
| | Retrospective | | |
| **Describe design:** | | | |

## 4. Sampling

**a. Sample included: (check all that apply)**

☐ Children/youth (ages 5–18)  ☐ Parents  ☐ School personnel  ☐ Community personnel

☐ Classroom  ☐ School  ☐ Community  ☐ Household

☐ Other. Please describe:

**b. Describe how each sample was obtained:**

**c. What was the sampling frame for each sample?**

**d. Study inclusion criteria for each sample:**

**e. Type of sample: (check all that apply and note for which sample)**

| Probability | Nonprobability |
|---|---|
| ☐ Simple random sampling | ☐ Convenience sampling |
| ☐ Stratified random sampling | ☐ Quota sampling |
| ☐ Cluster sampling | ☐ Purposive sampling |
| ☐ Census | ☐ Snowball sampling |
| ☐ Other. Please describe: | ☐ Other. Please describe: |

**f. What was the participation rate for each sample?**

Mark source of this rate:  ☐ Reported by authors  ☐ Calculated by the reviewer

**g. If the study was longitudinal, what were the retention rates by time period?**

☐ Mark here if the study was not longitudinal.

**h. Are there any selection bias issues mentioned and/or apparent?**    ☐ Yes    ☐ No

If yes, describe:

## 5. Sample Characteristics

| Children or Youth | N = | Other. Please describe: | N = |
|---|---|---|---|

| Age range:<br>Mean age:<br>Grade level in school: | Age range:<br>Mean age: |
|---|---|

**Socioeconomic status (describe how established as well):**

| Child gender:    % Male    % Female | Other gender:    % Male    % Female |
|---|---|

| Youth Race/Ethnicity: | Other Race/Ethnicity: |
|---|---|
| ____% American Indian or Alaska Native<br>____% Asian<br>____% Black or African American<br>____% Hispanic<br>____% Native Hawaiian or Other Pacific Islander<br>____% White<br>____% Other. Please describe:<br>____% Alternate Category. Please describe: | ____% American Indian or Alaska Native<br>____% Asian<br>____% Black or African American<br>____% Hispanic<br>____% Native Hawaiian or Other Pacific Islander<br>____% White<br>____% Other. Please describe:<br>____% Alternate Category. Please describe: |

**Country of study:** ☐ USA ☐ Other. Please describe:

## 6. Setting

School (during school day). Specify grade levels served by school:

☐ Recess      ☐ Physical education class      ☐ Other:
☐ Classroom      ☐ Lunch time
☐ School-wide      ☐ Special event
                 (e.g., jog-a-thon)

Before school (on school grounds or on the way to school):

After school (on school grounds). Specify grade levels served by school:

Community-based organization:

Other. Please describe:

**7. Theory and theoretical model as stated by author, if specified** (Is there a theoretical base for the study? If so, what theory is described? What are the relational forms in the model?)

**8. Describe the intervention conditions as stated by the author. Include a description of the structure (e.g., number of sessions, number of sessions per week, average length of each session, who is implementing and how those individuals are trained), topics covered and implementation:**

## 9a. Methods for Independent Variables As Reported by Authors (please use a separate row for each broad concept)

| Broad Concept or Construct | How Is Concept Operational-ized and for What Target Population (i.e., Indicators)? | Name of Scale or Index | # Items in Scale | Item and Summary Measurement Types (e.g., Nominal, Ordinal, Interval, Ratio) | Data Collection Method (e.g., Paper-Pencil Survey)[‡] | Informant or Information Source (e.g., Student, Teacher, Trained Data Collector)[§] | Data Collection Time Points[**] | Reliability Information (Note if from Study Sample or Other) | Validity Information (Note if from Study Sample or Other) |
|---|---|---|---|---|---|---|---|---|---|
| | | | | | | | | | |
| | | | | | | | | | |
| | | | | | | | | | |

[‡]The Access database will display a drop down box with the following response options: paper-pencil survey, computer assisted survey, fitness test, skill assessment, measurement device (e.g., pedometer, accelerometer, heart rate monitor), diary or journal, observation, interview, focus group, and other.

[§]The Access database will display a drop down box with the following options: student, teacher, parent, school administration, research staff, other adult, peer, and other.

[**]The Access database will display check boxes with the following response options: baseline, 1 month, 2 months, 3 months, 6 months, 12 months, 18 months, 24 months, 36 months, and other.

**9b. Methods for Dependent Variables As Reported by Authors** (please use a separate row for each broad concept)

| Broad Concept or Construct | How Is Concept Operational-ized and for What Target Population (i.e., Indicators)? | Name of Scale or Index | # Items in Scale | Item and Summary Measurement Types (e.g., Nominal, Ordinal, Interval, Ratio) | Data Collection Method (e.g., Paper-Pencil Survey)[††] | Informant or Information Source (e.g., Student, Teacher, Trained Data Collector)[‡‡] | Data Collection Time Points[§§] | Reliability Information (Note if from Study Sample or Other) | Validity Information (Note if from Study Sample or Other) |
|---|---|---|---|---|---|---|---|---|---|
| | | | | | | | | | |
| | | | | | | | | | |
| | | | | | | | | | |
| | | | | | | | | | |

[††]The Access database will display a drop down box with the following response options: paper-pencil survey, computer assisted survey, fitness test, skill assessment, measurement device (e.g., pedometer, accelerometer, heart rate monitor), diary or journal, observation, interview, focus group, and other.

[‡‡]The Access database will display a drop down box with the following options: student, teacher, parent, school administration, research staff, other adult, peer, and other.

[§§]The Access database will display check boxes with the following response options: baseline, 1 month, 2 months, 3 months, 6 months, 12 months, 18 months, 24 months, 36 months, and other.

## 10. Analytic strategy

**a. Describe the analytic strategy as stated by author (by outcome as appropriate):**

**b. Describe the covariates used for each analysis, as applicable:**

**c. Did the authors:**

| | Yes | No | NA | INP*** |
|---|---|---|---|---|
| Conduct statistical testing when appropriate? | Yes | No | NA | INP*** |
| Control for design effects in the statistical model (e.g., control for cluster design and/or repeated measures over time)? | Yes | No | NA | INP |
| Correct for multiple testing (e.g., Bonferroni or more stringent $p$-value)? | Yes | No | NA | INP |
| Experiments: Control for differential exposure to the intervention (dose)? | Yes | No | NA | INP |

**d. Missing data (describe how it was handled if applicable, e.g., listwise deletions, imputations):**

**e. Are there any other apparent problems with the data analyses?**     Yes     No     Not sure

If yes, please explain:

---

***INP=Information not provided.

## 11. Results

| Research Question or Hypothesis | Outcome or Broad Concept Tested | Results by Concept/ Outcome (Descriptive) | Results by Concept/ Outcome (Data Results) | N | Summary Include Magnitude of Association if Reported (e.g., effect size) | | Do Results Directly Relate to Paper Focus?[†††] |
|---|---|---|---|---|---|---|---|
| | | | | | Type of Association[‡‡‡] | Description of Association if Available | |
| | | | | | | | |
| | | | | | | | |
| | | | | | | | |

[†††]Please rate on a 3-point scale (0=No, not related; 1=Yes, a little; 2=Yes, a lot).
[‡‡‡]Please rate on a 3-point scale (0=Negative association, 1=No association, 2=Positive association).

**12. Limitations: What limitations were reported by the authors (as stated by author)?**

**13. Limitations noted by reviewers, but not reported by authors:**

**14. What type of activity does the article deal with? (Mark all that apply.)**
☐ Physical education class
☐ Regular recess
☐ Lunch recess
☐ Classroom-based, but not physical education classes specifically
☐ General physical activity (school-based or nonschool-based)
☐ Sports or athletics
☐ Other (please specify):

**15. Additional Comments:**

# Appendix C: Glossary of Research Design Terms

**Case-study design**

A case study is an in-depth examination (often over time) of one or a small number of cases believed to represent a broader phenomenon;[87] it is usually, but not always, observational.[88] In this report, all case studies reported only qualitative data.

**Cross-sectional study**

A cross-sectional study is conducted at a single time point (often through a survey), with a sample believed to represent a cross section of the population of interest on relevant variables such as sex, age, education levels, etc. Cross-sectional studies can be used to determine whether two variables are associated but do not allow for the direct examination of the impact of time on such associations, a condition necessary to establish casuality.[88,89]

**Descriptive design**

Descriptive studies have the purpose of describing activities, events, or behaviors that have occurred in a given situation; their goal is often to create a "profile" of a phenomenon, program, or population as it exists.[90] Descriptive and inferential statistics may be used.[87] These studies differ from most quasi-experimental and experimental designs in that they do not control environments or expose subjects to different treatments and typically lack a control or comparison group, making it more difficult to account for the influence of extraneous factors.[87,88]

**Experimental design**

Experimental design is often considered the most rigorous of research designs and is frequently referred to as the gold-standard for establishing causality; in order for a study to be classified as experimental, it must include a control group and use random assignment to intervention and control groups.[91] Results may not generalize beyond the sample or conditions of the experiment.[87]

**Intervention**

An intervention is "a specific activity (or set of related activities) intended to change the knowledge, attitudes, beliefs, behaviors, or practices of individuals and populations to reduce their health risk. An intervention has distinct process and outcome objectives and a protocol outlining the steps for implementation."[92]

**Longitudinal study**

A longitudinal study is a study conducted over time of a variable or a group of subjects,[87] unlike a cross-sectional study. By collecting data at a minimum of two distinct points in time,[90] one advantage of longitudinal studies is that they allow for the direct observation of the impact of time on variable associations, a condition necessary to establish casuality.[88] The studies in this review had a wide range of time between the initial and final data collection points; in some, final data were collected immediately following interventions, and in others, final data were collected as many as 4 years after the initial data collection.

**Quasi-experimental design**

A quasi-experimental design is similar to an experimental design but lacks the important characteristic of random assignment to intervention and control or comparison groups.[93] Though not considered as rigorous as an experimental design, it is often considered the next best thing for establishing causality.

# Appendix D: School-Based Physical Education Summary Matrix

Articles describing quasi-experimental or experimental designs are highlighted in the table before the matrix for each setting. Not all studies used these designs.

| School Based Physical Education Studies Using Quasi Experimental or Experimental Design (Authors and Date Only) | |
| --- | --- |
| Bluechardt, M.H., Shephard, R.J. | 1995 |
| Budde, H., Voelcker-Rehage, C., Pietraßyk-Kendziorra, S., Ribeiro, P., Tidow, G. | 2008 |
| Dwyer, T., Blizzard, L., Dean, K. | 1996 |
| Ericsson, I. | 2008 |
| McNaughten, D., Gabbard, C. | 1993 |
| Milosis, D., Papaioannou, A.G. | 2007 |
| Pollatschek, J.L., O'Hagan, F.J. | 1989 |
| Raviv, S., Low, M. | 1990 |
| Sallis, J.F., McKenzie, T.L., Kolody, B., Lewis, M., Marshall, S., Rosengard, P. | 1999 |
| Tremarche, P.V., Robinson, E.M., Graham, L.B. | 2007 |
| Tuckman, B.W., Hinkle, J.S. | 1986 |

**Appendix D: Physical Education Class Summary Matrix**[§§§]

| Study Citation | Study Focus and Setting | Sample Characteristics | Study Design and Data Collection | Intervention Conditions | Key Outcomes and Results |
|---|---|---|---|---|---|
| Bluechardt MH, Shephard RJ[41]<br><br>Using an extracurricular physical activity program to enhance social skills<br><br>*Journal of Learning Disabilities* 1995;28(3): 160-169 | **Study focus:** Physical education class<br><br>**Description:** Extracurricular physical activity program and self-reported academic competence<br><br>**Setting:** School<br><br>**Country:** Southern Ontario, Canada | **Sample 1:** Youth<br>**N:** 45<br><br>**Age range:** NR<br>**Mean age:** 9.4<br>**Grade:** Primary<br><br>**Gender:**<br>M: 76%<br>F: 24%<br><br>**Ethnicity:** NR | **Study design:** Experimental<br><br>**Data collection method and time points:**<br>Skill assessment (gross and fine motor skills as measured by Bruininks-Oseretsky Test of Motor Proficiency)<br>🕐 2 times (baseline, immediate follow-up after 10-week intervention)<br><br>Paper-pencil survey (self-report academic and non-academic competence, perception of physical and social performance during intervention as measured by the Self-Perception Profile for Learning Disabled Students)<br>🕐 2 times (baseline, 10 weeks)<br><br>Teacher observation (social behavior)<br>🕐 3 times (baseline, 10 weeks, 3 months) | **Conditions:** Students with learning disabilities participated in intense physical education instruction or academic enrichment.<br><br>**Structure:**<br>*Intervention:* Closely supervised twice-weekly, 90-minute extracurricular sessions in the pool or gymnasium designed to combine vigorous physical activity with social skills training and problem solving over a 10-week period. 26 instructors received 17 hours of training and were assigned 2 students each for the duration of the project.<br>*Control:* Students received the same amount of individual attention in academic instruction (twice weekly, 90 minutes, 10 weeks).<br><br>**Topics covered:**<br>*Intervention:* Gym sessions focused on upper-limb coordination (gross and fine motor). Pool sessions focused on strength and visual-motor control. Social skills were developed through modeling, practice problem-solving, role-play with feedback.<br>*Control:* Sessions focused on deficit skills as identified by classroom teacher.<br><br>**Methods:** Sessions were based on pool and gymnasium activities (one of each every week). 70 minutes of the 90 minutes were activity based. | **Does the intervention group perform significantly better on self-reported academic and teacher-observed social measures than the control group after 10-week intervention, controlling for gender?**[a]<br><br>• **Self-perception of general intellectual ability** — 0<br>• **Self-perception of spelling competence** — 0<br>• **Self-perception of mathematical competence** — 0<br>• **Self-perception of writing competence** — 0<br>• **Self-perception of reading competence** — 0<br>• **Global self-worth** — +<br>• Cooperates (social behavior) — 0<br>• Disrupts (social behavior) — 0<br>• Fights (social behavior) — 0<br>• Seeks help (social behavior) — 0<br>• Leader (social behavior) — 0<br><br>[a]Additional analyses showed that there were no significant group x time x gender effects on the outcomes.<br><br>**Does the intervention group perform significantly better on motor skills (as measured by Bruininks-Oseretsky Test of Motor Proficiency) and self-reported nonacademic measures than the control group after 10-week intervention, controlling for gender?**<br><br>• Composite motor skill scores (gross, fine, battery) — 0<br>• Nonacademic scores (social acceptance, athletic competence, physical appearance, behavioral conduct) — 0 |

[§§§]Results are coded as follows: + signifies a significant positive outcome; 0 signifies no significant outcome; – signifies a significant negative outcome. Matrices may not include all outcomes described in the article; shaded outcomes are outcomes of primary interest to (and were included in) this review; additional outcomes reported here may be of interest to readers.

NR = Not reported by study authors.

🕐 Indicates data collection time points.

| Study Citation | Study Focus and Setting | Sample Characteristics | Study Design and Data Collection | Intervention Conditions | Key Outcomes and Results |
|---|---|---|---|---|---|
| Budde H, Voelcker-Rehage C, Pietraßyk-Kendziorra S, Ribeiro P, Tidow G[49] Acute coordinative exercise improves attentional performance in adolescents. Neuroscience Letters 2008;441(2): 219-223 | Study focus: Physical education class Description: Effect of exercise on concentration and attention span Setting: School, physical education class Country: Germany | Sample 1: Youth N: 47 Age range: NR Mean age: 15.00 Grade: NR Gender: M: 76.60% F: 23.40% Ethnicity: NR Sample 2: Youth N: 52 Age range: NR Mean age:14.90 Grade: NR Gender: M: 84.60% F: 15.40% Ethnicity: NR | Study design: Experimental Data collection method and time points: Standardized tests (concentration and attention as measured by d2 test) ⏱ 2 times (pretest week 2 after a regular class and posttest week 3 after exercise or sport class) | Conditions: Students were assigned to the coordinated exercise condition or the normal sport lesson condition. Coordinated exercise condition (CE): Exercises selected from special forms for soccer and Munich Fitness test; groups of 4 students spent 1.75 minutes at each of 5 exercise stations. Normal sport lesson condition (NSL): Students exercised for 10 minutes at same intensity as CE group but without any specification on motor coordination. | Did the students in the coordinated exercise group have higher concentration and attention scores on the d2 test than control groups from pretest to posttest? • Overall concentration and attention + score Did the students in the coordinated exercise group have a greater number of correct responses on the d2 test than control groups from pretest to posttest? • Quantity of correct responses + • Quality of responses + Additional analyses showed that there were no significant effects of gender on the pretest to posttest changes. |
| Carlson SA, Fulton JE, Lee SM, Maynard LM, Brown DR, Kohl HW 3rd, et al.[52] Physical education and academic achievement in elementary school: data from the Early Childhood Longitudinal Study. American Journal of Public Health 2008;98(4): 721-727 | Study focus: Physical education class Description: Association between physical education and academic achievement Setting: School, physical education class, classroom Country: USA | Sample 1: Youth N: 5316 Age range: NR Mean age: 6.2 Grade: Primary (K–5th grades) Gender: M: 47.90% F: 52.10% Ethnicity: Hispanic: 13.3% White: 69.2% Other: 17.5% | Study design: Descriptive, secondary analysis of data from the Early Childhood Longitudinal Study, Kindergarten Class of 1998 to 1999 (ECLS-K) Data collection method and time points: Teacher report (times per week and minutes per day spent in physical education) ⏱ 5 times (baseline-Fall K, Spring K, Spring 1st, Spring 3rd, and Spring 5th grades) Standardized tests (math and reading item response theory [IRT] scores); ⏱ 5 times (baseline-Fall K, Spring K, Spring 1st, Spring 3rd, and Spring 5th grades) | No intervention | Do students who spend more time in physical education (medium vs. low physical education time) have higher academic achievement over time (as measured by IRT scores and controlling for demographics)? • Reading (boys) o • Reading (girls) o • Math (boys) o • Math (girls) o Do students who spend more time in physical education (high vs. low physical education time) have higher academic achievement over time (as measured by IRT scores and controlling for demographics)? • Reading (boys) o • Reading (girls) + o • Math (boys) o • Math (girls) + |

| Study Citation | Study Focus and Setting | Sample Characteristics | Study Design and Data Collection | Intervention Conditions | Key Outcomes and Results |
|---|---|---|---|---|---|
| Dexter T[53]<br><br>Relationships between sport knowledge, sport performance and academic ability: empirical evidence from GCSE Physical Education.<br><br>*Journal of Sports Sciences* 1999;17(4): 283-295 | **Study focus:** Physical education class<br><br>**Description:** The relationships between sport knowledge, sport performance, and academic ability<br><br>**Setting:** School, physical education class, classroom<br><br>**Country:** UK | **Sample 1:** Youth<br>**N:** 517<br>**Age range:** NR<br>**Mean age:** 16.00<br>**Grade:** Secondary (at completion of compulsory school)<br>**Gender:** NR<br>**Ethnicity:** NR | **Study design:** Descriptive, secondary analysis of data from the 1995 General Certificate of Secondary Education (GCSE) examination in physical education, math, and English<br><br>**Data collection method and time points:** Standardized tests (GCSE/English, math, physical education knowledge, sport knowledge)<br>🕐 1 time<br><br>Skill assessment (badminton, basketball, football, hockey, rounders, netball, average sport performance score as measured by Amateur Athletic Association ESSO 5 Star points system)<br>🕐 1 time | No intervention | Is academic ability (as measured by GCSE English scores) associated with sport skill performance (assessed by teachers)?[b]<br>- Football +<br>- Badminton +<br>- Basketball 0<br>- Hockey +<br>- Netball +<br>- Rounders 0<br>- Athletics +<br><br>Is academic ability (as measured by GCSE math scores) associated with sport skill performance (as assessed by teachers)?[b]<br>- Football +<br>- Badminton +<br>- Basketball 0<br>- Hockey +<br>- Netball +<br>- Rounders +<br>- Athletics +<br><br>[b]Additional analyses by gender showed similar results. |
| Dollman J, Boshoff K, Dodd G[54]<br><br>The relationship between curriculum time for physical education and literacy and numeracy standards in South Australian primary schools.<br><br>*European Physical Education Review* 2006;12(2): 151-163 | **Study focus:** Physical education class<br><br>**Description:** The relationship between curriculum time for physical education and literacy and numeracy standards in South Australian primary schools.<br><br>**Setting:** School<br><br>**Country:** Australia | **Sample 1:** School<br>**N:** 117<br>**Grade:** Primary and Secondary (3rd, 5th and 7th grades) | **Study design:** Descriptive<br><br>**Data collection method and time points:** Principal paper-pencil survey (curriculum time dedicated to physical education, physical education staff age and physical education training, ethnicity, SES)<br>🕐 1 time<br><br>Standardized tests (state literacy and numeracy tests—State LaN)<br>🕐 2 times (baseline, 12 months) | No intervention | Does curriculum time committed to physical education independently predict literacy and numeracy competencies assessed by the State Literacy and Numeracy Test (controlling for socioeconomic status (SES), nonEnglish-speaking background, and staff profile variables)?<br>- Literacy 0<br>- Numeracy 0<br>- Average school attainment in both literacy and numeracy 0 |

| Study Citation | Study Focus and Setting | Sample Characteristics | Study Design and Data Collection | Intervention Conditions | Key Outcomes and Results |
|---|---|---|---|---|---|
| Dwyer T, Blizzard L, Dean K[42]<br><br>Physical activity and performance in children.<br><br>*Nutrition Reviews* 1996;54(4 Pt 2):S27-S31 | **Study focus:** Physical education class<br><br>**Description:** Physical activity and academic performance<br><br>**Setting:** School, classroom<br><br>**Country:** Australia<br><br>*This article also reported on the Australian School Health and Fitness Study (ASHFS); those data are not presented here because they did not meet inclusion criteria.* | **Sample 1:** School N: 7<br>**Grade:** Primary (5th grade)<br><br>**Sample 2:** Youth N: 501<br>**Age range:** NR<br>**Mean age:** 10<br>**Grade:** Primary (5th grade)<br>**Gender:** NR<br>**Ethnicity:** NR | **Study design:** Experimental<br><br>**Data collection method and time points:** Observation (classroom behavior)<br>⏱ 2 times (baseline, 1 week post intervention)<br><br>Measurement device (height and weight, skinfold test, endurance fitness test)<br>⏱ 2 times (baseline, 1 week post intervention)<br><br>Standardized tests (the Australian Council for Educational Research arithmetic test and the GAP reading test)<br>⏱ 2 times (baseline, 1 week post intervention) | **Name:** School Health, Academic Performance and Exercise (SHAPE) study<br><br>**Structure:** Students were divided into three groups (skill, fitness, and control) that focused on developing student skill and competence level in minor games. The intervention took place over 14 weeks and was overseen by the investigators to ensure adherence.<br><br>**Implementation:** In the skill group, the exercise (duration and frequency) was increased to 75 minutes daily, 15 minutes of which were in the morning. The fitness group had the same. | **Does participation in a fitness program improve performance on arithmetic and reading tests?**<br>• Academic performance   0<br><br>**Does participation in a fitness program improve classroom behavior (as observed by teacher)?**<br>• Classroom behavior   +<br><br>**Does participation in a fitness program improve measures of Physical Work Capacity and BMI?**<br>• Physical work capacity (fitness)   +<br>• Skinfold sum scores   + |
| Ericsson I[43]<br><br>Motor skills, attention and academic achievements: an intervention study in school years 1-3.<br><br>*British Educational Research Journal* 2008;34(3): 301-313 | **Study focus:** Physical education class<br><br>**Description:** Motor skills and attention and academic achievement<br><br>**Setting:** School, physical education class<br><br>**Country:** Sweden | **Sample 1:** Youth N: 251<br>**Age range:** 7-9<br>**Mean age:** NR<br>**Grade:** Primary (1st-3rd grades)<br>**Gender:**<br>M: 55%<br>F: 45%<br>**Ethnicity:** NR | **Study design:** Quasi-experimental<br><br>**Data collection method and time points:** Skill assessment using the Motorisk Utveckling som Grund för Inlärning (MUGI) checklist (observation of 16 gross motor tasks measuring balance/bilateral coordination and hand-eye coordination) in 2nd and 3rd grades<br>⏱ 3 times, data collection timepoints varied by cohort (baseline, year 2, year 3)<br><br>Paper-pencil survey using Conners' questionnaire (teachers' and parents' conception of children's attention ability and impulse control) | **Conditions:**<br>*Intervention:* Students received physical education lessons 5 days per week.<br>*Comparison:* Standard physical education lessons 2 days per week.<br><br>**Methods:**<br>*Intervention:* 3 regular school physical education lessons per week plus different local sports clubs gave physical activity lessons for 2 more lessons every week, for a total of 5 lessons of motor skills training and physical activity per week. If needed (for students deemed motor deficient), 1 extra lesson of MUGI motor training per week was provided. | **Do students with good motor skills have better attention than students with deficits in motor skills (as observed by teachers and parents)?**<br>• Attention   +<br>• Impulse control   +<br><br>**Do students in intervention groups have better attention than students in comparison group (as observed by teachers and parents)?**<br>• Attention 2nd grade   +<br>• Impulse control 2nd grade   +<br>• Attention 3rd grade   0<br>• Impulse control 3rd grade   0<br><br>**Do students in intervention groups have better standardized test scores than students in comparison group?** |

| Study Citation | Study Focus and Setting | Sample Characteristics | Study Design and Data Collection | Intervention Conditions | Key Outcomes and Results |
|---|---|---|---|---|---|
| | | | ⟳ 3 times (baseline, year 2, year 3)<br><br>Standardized tests (special education teachers document reading development in 1st and 2nd grades)<br><br>⟳ 3 times (baseline, 6 months, 18 months)<br><br>Standardized tests (national tests in Swedish, math, words, reading)<br><br>⟳ 1 time (Swedish and math: Spring of 2nd grade; words and reading: Spring of 3rd grade) | | • **Swedish reading and writing** +<br>• **Math (spatial ability and number conception)**[c] +<br><br>Do children's observed motor skills improve with extended physical activity and extra motor training in school?[c]<br>• **Motor skills**[d] +<br><br>[c]Additional analyses by gender showed that intervention boys had significantly better math scores than control boys.<br>[d]After 1 year, differences between groups were rather large (0.24), and in year 3, differences were very large (0.37). |
| McNaughton D, Gabbard C[44]<br><br>Physical exertion and immediate mental performance of sixth-grade children.<br><br>*Perceptual and Motor Skills* 1993;77(3 Pt 2):1155-1159 | **Study focus:** Physical education class<br><br>**Description:** Physical exertion and mathematical performance<br><br>**Setting:** School, classroom<br><br>**Country:** USA | **Sample 1:** Youth<br>**N:** 120<br>**Age range:** NR<br>**Mean age:** 11.3<br>**Grade:** Secondary (6th grade)<br>**Gender:**<br>M: 50%<br>F: 50%<br>**Ethnicity:** NR | **Study design:** Experimental<br><br>**Data collection method and time points:** Measurement device (time of day and duration of walking activity)<br>⟳ 11 times (baseline, Tuesday, Wednesday, Thursday of week 2, 3, 4 and Tuesday of week 5)<br><br>Mathematical test<br>⟳ 11 times (baseline, Tuesday, Wednesday, Thursday of week 2, 3, 4 and Tuesday of week 5) | **Structure:** Two procedures: walking for a specific duration and receiving a timed mathematical computation test. Testing was conducted over a 5-week period.<br><br>**Methods:** Subjects walked around the perimeter of a regulation basketball court at a monitored moderate intensity (120 to 145 beats per minute). Walking duration was systematically ordered for the 20, 30, and 40 minutes. Walking occurred early morning (8:30 a.m.), before lunch (11:50 a.m.) or afternoon (2:20 p.m.). A mathematics test was given at the end of the specified duration of activity, and subjects had 90 seconds to complete the task. | **Does increased duration (20, 30 or 40 minutes) of physical exertion (walking) lead to improved mathematical test scores?**<br><br>• **Math test score (20 minutes)** 0<br>• **Math test score (30 minutes)** +<br>• **Math test score (40 minutes)** +<br><br>**Does the time of day[e] and duration of student exposure to physical activity (walking) improve math performance?**<br><br>• **Math test score (morning)** 0<br>• **Math test score (before lunch)** +<br>• **Math test score (after lunch)** +<br><br>[e]Additional analyses showed that gender did not have a significant effect or interaction with the results. |

| Study Citation | Study Focus and Setting | Sample Characteristics | Study Design and Data Collection | Intervention Conditions | Key Outcomes and Results |
|---|---|---|---|---|---|
| Milosis D, Papaioannou AG[47]<br><br>Interdisciplinary teaching, multiple goals and self-concept.<br><br>In: Liukkonen J, Vanden Auweele Y, Vereijken B, Alfermann D, Theodorakis Y, editors. *Psychology for Physical Educators: Student in Focus.* 2nd edition. Champaign, IL: Human Kinetics; 2007:175-198 | **Study focus:** Physical education class<br><br>**Description:** The effect of an interdisciplinary approach to teaching physical education on self-concept and goals<br><br>**Setting:** School, physical education class<br><br>**Country:** Greece | **Sample 1:** Youth<br>**N:** 292<br>**Age range:** NR<br>**Mean age:** 12.3<br>**Grade:** Initial grade in Greek junior high school<br>**Gender:**<br>**M:** 55%<br>**F:** 45% | **Study design:** Experimental<br><br>**Data collection method and time points:** Paper-pencil survey (self-concept)<br>🕒 2 times (baseline, 6 months)<br><br>Administrative records (math and Greek language grades)<br>🕒 2 times (baseline, 9 months) | **Name:** Multidimensional Model of Goal Orientations (MMGO)<br><br>**Conditions:** Students participated in the MMGO physical education curriculum or standard physical education class.<br><br>**Structure:**<br>*Intervention:* MMGO physical education class taught 3 times per week for 6 months by specially trained physical education teacher.<br>*Control:* Standard physical education class 3 times per week for 6 months.<br><br>**Topics covered:** The MMGO course focused on personal improvement goals and outcomes in the health domain, the achievement domain, and the social domain. | Does student participation in the MMGO intervention improve math and language grades, student reported self-concept, and life satisfaction?<br>• General self-concept + <br>• General school self-concept + <br>• Mathematics self-concept + <br>• Greek language self-concept + <br>• Math grades 0 <br>• Language grades + <br>• Life satisfaction + |
| Pollatschek JL, O'Hagan FJ[45]<br><br>An investigation of the psycho-physical influences of a quality daily physical education programme.<br><br>*Health Education Research* 1989;4(3):341-350 | **Study focus:** Physical education class<br><br>**Description:** Effect of daily physical education vs. physical education twice a week on physical, academic, and affective student outcomes<br><br>**Setting:** School, physical education class<br><br>**Country:** Scotland | **Sample 1:** School<br>**N:** 399<br>**Age range:** NR<br>**Mean age:** NR<br>**Grade:** Secondary (6th grade) | **Study design:** Quasi-experimental<br><br>**Data collection method and time points:** Paper-pencil survey (attitude towards school and school work, social relations, and personality)<br>🕒 2 times (baseline, end of academic year)<br><br>Fitness test (motor fitness: muscular strength and endurance, circulatory endurance, muscular power, agility, flexibility, and speed as measured by Canadian Association of Health, Physical Education and Recreation (CAHPER) Fitness-Performance II Test)<br>🕒 2 times (baseline, end of academic year)<br><br>Standardized tests (reading, math 'GAPADOL')<br>🕒 2 times (baseline, end of academic year) | **Conditions:**<br>*Intervention:* Students participated in daily physical education.<br>*Comparison:* 2 periods of physical education per week.<br><br>**Methods:**<br>*Intervention:* Daily PE classes usually consisting of 45 to 60 minutes per day but as much as half a day on certain activities, such as orienteering. | Was the daily physical education program associated with improved performance scores (standardized test scores and self-reported attitude) compared with standard physical education?[f]<br>• Math scores 0 <br>• Reading scores 0 <br>• Attitude toward school 0 <br><br>[f]Additional analyses showed that gender did not have a significant effect on academic achievement.<br><br>Was the daily physical education program associated with improved motor fitness scores compared with standard physical education?[g]<br>• Motor fitness (girls) + <br>• Motor fitness (boys) + <br><br>[g]Intervention girls scored higher on every motor fitness test; intervention boys scored higher on shuttle run and 50-meter run. |

| Study Citation | Study Focus and Setting | Sample Characteristics | Study Design and Data Collection | Intervention Conditions | Key Outcomes and Results |
|---|---|---|---|---|---|
| Raviv S, Low M[46]<br><br>Influence of physical activity on concentration among junior high-school students.<br><br>*Perceptual and Motor Skills* 1990;70(1):67-74 | **Study focus:** Physical education class<br><br>**Description:** Physical education and concentration<br><br>**Setting:** School, physical education class, classroom<br><br>**Country:** Israel | **Sample 1:** Youth<br>**N:** 96<br>**Age range:** 11–12<br>**Mean age:** NR<br>**Grade:** Secondary (Israeli junior high school)<br>**Gender:** NR<br>**Ethnicity:** NR | **Study design:** Quasi-experimental<br><br>**Data collection method and time points:** Standardized tests (concentration as measured by d2 test)<br>🕐 NR | **Conditions:** Students were divided into 4 groups: 2 participated in physical education class and 2 studied science.<br><br>**Structure:** Each subject was taught twice a day by the same teacher at the beginning and end of the school day. | **Does course content (science or physical education) improve student levels of concentration measured by the d2 test?**<br>• **Better concentration in science than physical education**  0<br><br>**Does timing (beginning or end of class) improve student levels of concentration measured by the d2 test?**<br>• Better concentration at the ends of lessons than the beginning  +<br>• Better concentration at the beginning of the day than the end of the day  + |
| Sallis JF, McKenzie TL, Kolody B, Lewis M, Marshall S, Rosengard P[48]<br><br>Effects of health-related physical education on academic achievement: Project SPARK.<br><br>*Research Quarterly for Exercise and Sport* 1999;70(2):127-134 | **Study Focus:** Physical education class<br><br>**Description:** The effect of school physical education on standardized test scores<br><br>**Setting:** School day, physical education class, classroom<br><br>**Country:** USA | **Sample 1:** Schools<br>**N:** 7<br><br>**Sample 2:** Youth<br>**N:** 759<br>**Age range:** NR<br>**Mean age:** 9.5<br>**Grade:** Primary (4th–6th grade)<br>**Gender:**<br>M: 52%<br>F: 48%<br>**Ethnicity:**<br>Black: 2.2%<br>Hispanic: 4.9%<br>Asian/Pacific Islander: 14.2% | **Study design:** Experimental<br><br>**Data collection method and time points:** Paper-pencil survey (standardized test in reading, language, math, and basic battery as measured by Metropolitan Achievement test—MAT6 and MAT7)<br>🕐 2 times (baseline in 2nd grade, cohort 1 in Spring of 5th grade, cohort 2 in Fall of 6th grade) | **Name:** SPARK (physical education curriculum)<br><br>**Conditions:** Students were assigned to SPARK physical education classes taught by physical education specialists, by trained classroom teachers, or standard physical education (control).<br><br>**Structure:** Four 30-minute lessons total per week: 3 days of physical education lessons including health-fitness and skill-fitness activities plus 30 minutes of classroom lesson on behavior change/self-management.<br><br>**Topics covered:** 13 health-fitness units and 9 sports units<br><br>**Methods:** Brief review of skills, presentation of new topic, set physical activity goals. | **Did exposure to SPARK physical education improve student outcomes on standardized tests?**<br><br>**Reading**<br>• Cohort 1  +<br>• Cohort 2  +<br>**Math**<br>• Cohort 1  0<br>• Cohort 2  0<br>**Language**<br>• Cohort 1  +<br>• Cohort 2  -<br>**Basic battery**<br>• Cohort 1  0<br>• Cohort 2  + |

| Study Citation | Study Focus and Setting | Sample Characteristics | Study Design and Data Collection | Intervention Conditions | Key Outcomes and Results |
|---|---|---|---|---|---|
| Tremarche PV, Robinson EM, Graham LB[51]<br><br>Physical education and its effect on elementary testing results.<br><br>*Physical Educator* 2007;64(2):58-64 | **Study focus:** Physical education class<br><br>**Description:** The impact of increased quality physical education time on standardized test scores<br><br>**Setting:** School<br><br>**Country:** USA | **Sample 1:** Youth<br>**N:** 311<br>**Age range:** 9-11<br>**Mean age:** NR<br>**Grade:** Primary (4th grade)<br>**Gender:** NR<br>**Ethnicity:**<br>**Indian:** 3.3%<br>**Asian:** .6%<br>**Black:** 2.6%<br>**Hispanic:** 1%<br>**White:** 92.5% | **Study design:** Quasi-experimental<br><br>**Data collection method and time points:** Standardized tests (English and language arts and math on the Massachusetts Comprehensive Assessment System—MCAS scores)<br>⏰ 1 time<br><br>Paper-pencil survey (student time in physical education per school year)<br>⏰ 1 time | No intervention | **Did students who received more hours of physical education score higher on the MCAS test?**<br><br>• English language arts    +<br>• Math    0 |
| Tuckman BW, Hinkle JS[50]<br><br>An experimental study of the physical and psychological effects of aerobic exercise on schoolchildren.<br><br>*Health Psychology* 1986;5(3):197-207 | **Study focus:** Physical education class<br><br>**Description:** Physical and psychological effects of aerobic exercise<br><br>**Setting:** School, physical education class<br><br>**Country:** USA | **Sample 1:** Youth<br>**N:** 154<br>**Age range:** 9.30-11.30<br>**Mean age:** NR<br>**Grade:** Cross level (4th-6th grades)<br>**Gender:** NR<br>**Ethnicity:**<br>Nonwhite: 27-29% | **Study design:** Experimental<br><br>**Data collection method and time points:** Measurement device (time on 50-meter run)<br>⏰ 2 times<br><br>Measurement device (time on 800-meter run)<br>⏰ 3 times (baseline, posttest, 5 months after posttest)<br><br>Measurement device (skinfold test for body fat, pulse rate)<br>⏰ 2 times<br><br>Paper-pencil survey (teacher rating of student behavior as conducive or disruptive to classroom participation)<br>⏰ 2 times<br><br>Skill assessment (perceptual-motor ability as measured by Bender-Gestalt test)<br>⏰ 2 times | **Conditions:** Students participated in the running program or regular physical education.<br><br>**Structure:**<br>*Intervention:* 3 running sessions per week for 12 weeks. Each session lasted 30 minutes. The sessions were conducted by the research team as part of students' physical education classes.<br>*Control:* regular physical education program, which included basketball, volleyball, and occasional jogging. Regular physical education took place 3 times per week for 6th-grade students and 5 times per week for 4th- and 5th-grade students.<br><br>**Methods:** The running took place on a 400-meter track and consisted of gradual increments in distance, interval workouts, and relay runs. | **Does exposure to the intervention improve children's physical and psychological outcomes?**<br><br>• Creativity (Alternate Uses test)    +<br>• Classroom behavior (teacher observation)    +<br>• Perceived self-concept (self-report)    0<br>• Perceptual motor ability (Bender-Gestalt test)    0<br>• Planning ability and visual-motor coordination (Maze Tracing test)    0<br><br>Additional analyses of treatment x gender showed no differences for classroom behavior, self-concept, Bender-Gestalt test. However, treatment boys and treatment girls performed better on the maze test than control boys and control girls, respectively.<br><br>**Does exposure to the intervention improve children's physical outcomes?** |

| Study Citation | Study Focus and Setting | Sample Characteristics | Study Design and Data Collection | Intervention Conditions | Key Outcomes and Results |
|---|---|---|---|---|---|
| | | | Skill assessment (planning ability and visual motor coordination as measured by the Maze Tracing Test) ↻ 2 times<br><br>Paper-pencil survey (creativity as measured by the Alternative Uses Test measuring divergent thinking; self-concept as measured by Piers-Harris Children's Self-Concept Scale) ↻ 2 times | | • 800-meter run (boys and girls) +<br>• 800-meter run (5-month follow-up—boys) +<br>• 800-meter run (5-month follow-up—girls) 0<br>• 50-meter dash 0<br>• Pulse rate +<br>• Skinfold (body fat) (boys) +<br>• Skinfold (body fat) (girls) 0 |

# Appendix E: Recess Summary Matrix

Articles describing quasi-experimental or experimental designs are highlighted in the table before the matrix for each setting. Not all studies used these designs.

| Recess Studies Using Quasi Experimental or Experimental Design (Authors and Date Only) | |
|---|---|
| Caterino, M.C., Polak, E.D. | 1999 |
| Jarrett, O.S., Maxwell, D.M., Dickerson, C., Hoge, P., Davies, G., Yetley, A. | 1998 |
| Pellegrini, A.D., Davis, P.D. | 1993 |
| Pellegrini, A.D., Huberty, P.D., Jones, I. | 1995 |

**Appendix E: Recess Summary Matrix\*\*\***

| Study Citation | Study Focus and Setting | Sample Characteristics | Study Design and Data Collection | Intervention Conditions | Key Outcomes and Results |
|---|---|---|---|---|---|
| Barros, RM, Silver, EJ, Stein, REK[58]<br><br>School recess and group classroom behavior.<br><br>*Pediatrics* 2009; 123(2):431-436 | **Study focus:** Recess<br><br>**Description:** The effect of exposure to recess on primary school students' classroom behavior<br><br>**Setting:** School, recess<br><br>**Country:** USA | **Sample 1:** Youth<br>**N:** 11,529<br>**Age range:** 8–9<br>**Mean age:** NR<br>**Grade:** Primary (3rd grade)<br>**Gender:**<br>M: 50.3%<br>F: 49.7%<br><br>**Ethnicity:**<br>Black: 12%<br>Hispanic: 16%<br>Other/mixed: 11%<br>White: 61% | **Study design:** Descriptive, secondary analysis of Early Childhood Longitudinal Study (ECLS) dataset (Kindergarten Class of 1998–1999)<br><br>**Data collection method and time points:** Paper-pencil survey (teacher report of frequency of recess and physical education class, classroom characteristics, and teacher rating of group classroom behavior)<br>🕐 1 time (students in 3rd grade) | No intervention | **Do students who are exposed to recess during the school day have better classroom behavior, as reported by the teacher, than students who do not have recess?** + <br><br>• **Classroom behavior (overall classroom)**<br><br>Results were also examined by the level of exposure to recess. All levels of recess showed significantly better classroom behavior when compared with no recess. Differences were not significant between exposure levels.<br><br>Additional analyses by ethnicity and SES revealed significant differences. Black and Hispanic students and lower income students were all significantly less likely to have recess. There were no differences by gender. |
| Caterino MC, Polak ED[55]<br><br>Effects of two types of activity on the performance of second-, third-, and fourth-grade students on a test of concentration.<br><br>*Perceptual and Motor Skills* 1999; 89(1):245-248 | **Study focus:** Recess<br><br>**Description:** The effect of physical activity on elementary school students' concentration<br><br>**Setting:** School, classroom, library and gym<br><br>**Country:** USA | **Sample 1:** Youth<br>**N:** 54<br>**Age range:** NR<br>**Mean age:** NR<br>**Grade:** Primary (3rd, 4th, and 5th grades)<br>**Gender:** NR<br>**Ethnicity:** NR<br><br>**Sample 2:** Youth<br>**N:** 71<br>**Mean age:** NR<br>**Grade:** Primary<br>**Gender:** NR<br>**Ethnicity:** NR<br><br>**Sample 3:** Youth<br>**N:** 52<br>**Mean age:** NR<br>**Grade:** Primary<br>**Gender:** NR<br>**Ethnicity:** NR | **Study design:** Experimental<br><br>**Data collection method and time points:** Standardized tests (concentration as measured by the Woodcock-Johnson Test of Concentration)<br>🕐 1 time (immediately after intervention) | **Conditions:** Physical activity group, classroom activity group<br><br>**Structure:** Students in the physical activity group went to the gym for 15 minutes of stretching and aerobic walking and then to the library for the Woodcock-Johnson Test of Concentration. Students in the classroom activity group participated in regular classroom activities and then went to the library for the Woodcock-Johnson Test of Concentration. | **Do students who participate in directed physical activity have significantly higher scores on the Woodcock-Johnson Test of Concentration than students who participate in typical classroom activity?** + <br><br>• **Concentration (4th-grade students)** |

\*\*\*Results are coded as follows: + signifies a significant positive outcome; 0 signifies no significant outcome; – signifies a significant negative outcome. Matrices may not include all outcomes described in the article; shaded outcomes are outcomes of primary interest to (and were included in) this review; additional outcomes reported here may be of interest to readers.

NR=Not reported by study authors.

🕐 Indicates data collection time points.

| Study Citation | Study Focus and Setting | Sample Characteristics | Study Design and Data Collection | Intervention Conditions | Key Outcomes and Results |
|---|---|---|---|---|---|
| Jarrett OS, Maxwell DM, Dickerson C, Hoge P, Davies G, Yetley A[56]<br><br>Impact of recess on classroom behavior: Group effects and individual differences.<br><br>*Journal of Educational Research* 1998; 92(2):121-126 | **Study focus:** Recess<br><br>**Description:** The effect of recess on classroom behavior<br><br>**Setting:** School, recess, classroom<br><br>**Country:** USA | **Sample 1:** Youth<br>**N:** 43<br>**Age range:** NR<br>**Mean age:** NR<br>**Grade:** Primary (4th grade)<br>**Gender:**<br>M: 41.9%<br>F: 58.1%<br>**Ethnicity:**<br>Black: 18.6%<br>White: 81.4% | **Study design:** Quasi-experimental<br><br>**Data collection method and time points:** Observation (classroom behavior: concentration, fidgety, work, listless)<br>⏱ 6 times (baseline [mid-November] to mid-March [until 6 recesses per child])<br><br>Observation (academic achievement)<br>⏱ 1 time (year-end) | **Structure:** Children were observed in the classroom each week on the 2 days that they did not have physical education. During the first week of observation, each class was randomly assigned to have recess on one of the days and no recess on the other day (recess amounted to 15 to 20 minutes). | **Does recess improve students' on-task behavior and decrease students' fidgetiness in the classroom (as observed by research staff)?**<br>• On-task behavior +<br>• Less fidgetiness + |
| Pellegrini AD, Davis PD[57]<br><br>Relations between children's playground and classroom behaviour.<br><br>*British Journal of Educational Psychology* 1993; 63(1):88-95 | **Study focus:** Recess<br><br>**Description:** Relationships between children's playground and classroom behavior<br><br>**Setting:** School, recess<br><br>**Country:** USA | **Sample 1:** School<br>**N:** 1<br>**Grade:** Primary (3rd grade)<br><br>**Sample 2:** Youth<br>**N:** 23<br>**Age range:** NR<br>**Mean age:** 9.4<br>**Grade:** Primary (3rd grade)<br>**Gender:**<br>M: 60.9%<br>F: 39.1%<br>**Ethnicity:** NR | **Study design:** Quasi-experimental<br><br>**Data collection method and time points:** Standardized Test (cognitive ability as measured by the Iowa Test of Basic Skills (1986))<br>⏱ 1 time<br><br>Observation (concentration and fidgeting in classroom and nonsocial exercise, social exercise, nonsocial sedentary, and social sedentary recess behavior)<br>⏱ 32 times (only when outdoor play time occurred during the 14-week data collection period) | **Conditions:** Students were exposed to 1 of 2 conditions, a shorter confinement period in the classroom (2.5 hours) and a longer confinement period in the classroom (3 hours) before recess.<br><br>**Structure:** Each child was exposed to both conditions by counterbalancing the order in which the whole class experienced confinement across the 14-week observation period.<br><br>**Method:** Students were observed before recess, during recess, and after recess. | **Does children's observed exercise behavior (social and nonsocial)[h] during recess improve observed classroom behavior immediately following recess (controlling for standardized test scores)?**<br>• Fidget (social exercise behavior) +<br>• Fidget (nonsocial exercise behavior) +<br><br>**Does children's observed sedentary behavior (social and nonsocial)[h] during recess improve observed classroom behavior immediately following recess (controlling for standardized test scores)?**<br>• Fidget (social sedentary behavior) –<br>• Concentration (social sedentary behavior) +<br>• Concentration (nonsocial sedentary behavior) –<br><br>[h] *Social exercise behavior:* Children were exchanging language, gestures, or gazes while engaging in gross body and/or muscular activity. *Nonsocial exercise behavior:* gross body and/or muscular activity alone or without interacting with others. *Social sedentary behavior:* Nonstrenuous exercise such as walking, sitting, or standing while interacting with others. *Nonsocial sedentary behavior:* nonstrenuous exercise without interacting with others. |

| Study Citation | Study Focus and Setting | Sample Characteristics | Study Design and Data Collection | Intervention Conditions | Key Outcomes and Results |
|---|---|---|---|---|---|
| Pellegrini AD, Huberty PD, Jones J[37]<br><br>The effects of recess timing on children's playground and classroom behaviors.<br><br>American Educational Research Journal 1995;32(4):845-864 | **Study focus:** Recess<br><br>**Description:** Recess and its impact on student behavior in the classroom and on the playground<br><br>**Setting:** School, recess<br><br>**Country:** USA | **Sample 1:** Youth<br>N: 37<br>**Age range:** NR<br>**Mean age:** NR<br>**Grade:** Primary (2nd, 4th grades)<br>**Gender:**<br>M: 46%<br>F: 54%<br>**Ethnicity:**<br>Black: 30.0%<br>White: 70.0%<br><br>**Sample 2:** Youth<br>N: 62<br>**Age range:** NR<br>**Mean age:** 7.6<br>**Grade:** Primary (K, 2nd, 4th grades)<br>**Gender:**<br>M: 55.0%<br>F: 45.0%<br>**Ethnicity:**<br>Black: 30.0%<br>White: Majority %<br>Asian: Small %<br><br>**Sample 3:** Youth<br>N: 44<br>**Age range:** NR<br>**Mean age:** 10.1<br>**Grade:** Primary (4th grade)<br>**Gender:**<br>M: 39.0%<br>F: 61.0%<br>**Ethnicity:** NR | **Study design:** Quasi-experimental<br><br>**Data collection method and time points:** Observation (social interaction during recess, inattention before and after recess, physical activity during recess)<br>🕐 32 times (every Monday–Thursday for 2 months) | **Conditions:** Children in 2nd and 4th grades were presented with either a male-preferred or female-preferred task immediately before recess and immediately after recess. Children were expected to sit quietly in their seats while the teacher read a story with either a male or female main character.<br><br>**Structure:** 4 days per week recess timing was manipulated: 2 days per week students went to recess at 10:00 a.m. (short deprivation period) and 2 days per week students went to recess at 10:30 a.m. (long deprivation period).<br><br>**Method:** Students were observed before recess, during recess, and after recess. | **Are children more attentive to classroom tasks after recess than before recess (as observed by research staff)?**<br><br>**Experiment 1:**<br>• More attentive (grades 2 and 4)  +<br>• More attentive (K)  0<br><br>**Experiment 2:**<br>• More attentive (grade 2)  +<br>• More attentive (grade 4)  0<br><br>**Experiment 3:**<br>• More attentive (class 1)  +<br>• More attentive (class 2)  0<br><br>**Does children's observed behavior during recess affect post-recess classroom attention (as observed by research staff)?**<br><br>**Experiment 1:**<br>• Attention  0<br><br>**Experiment 2:**<br>• Attention  0<br><br>**Experiment 3:**<br>• Attention  0<br><br>**Does the timing of recess (after 2.5 or 3 hours of classroom time) affect the playground physical activity and social interaction (as observed by research staff)?**<br><br>Experiment 1:<br>• More physical activity  0<br>• More social interaction (4th-grade students)  +<br><br>Experiment 2:<br>• More physical activity (2nd- and 4th-grade students)  0<br>• More social interaction  +<br><br>Experiment 3:<br>• More physical activity (boys)  +<br>• More social interaction  0 |

| Study Citation | Study Focus and Setting | Sample Characteristics | Study Design and Data Collection | Intervention Conditions | Key Outcomes and Results |
|---|---|---|---|---|---|
| Pellegrini AD, Kato K, Blatchford P, Baines E[59]<br><br>A short-term longitudinal study of children's playground games across the first year of school: Implications for social competence and adjustment to school.<br><br>*American Educational Research Journal* 2002;39(4):991-1015 | **Study focus:** Recess<br><br>**Description:** School adjustment, game facilitation, play/games behaviors<br><br>**Setting:** School, recess<br><br>**Country:** USA | **Sample 1:** Youth<br>**N:** 77<br>**Age range:** NR<br>**Mean age:** 6.4<br>**Grade:** Primary (1st grade)<br>**Gender:**<br>**M:** 39.0%<br>**F:** 61.0%<br>**Ethnicity:** NR | **Study design:** Descriptive, with longitudinal follow-up<br><br>**Data collection method and time points:** Paper-pencil survey (teacher and researcher checklist of student behavior of adjustment to school, facility in sports and games)<br>⏱ 2 times (late Fall and early Spring)<br><br>Observation (student game behaviors and game facility)<br>⏱ 12 times (observed for minimum of 3 minutes per month)<br><br>Interview (peer nominations, school connectedness)<br>⏱ 2 times (early Fall and late Spring) | No intervention | **Does a composite measure of students' "game facility"[a] predict end-of-year school adjustment (based on research staff and teacher aggregate ratings)?**<br><br>• School adjustment (boys) +<br>• School adjustment (girls) 0<br><br>Does a composite measure of game facility predict student's end-of-year social competence (based on research staff and teacher aggregate ratings)?<br><br>• Social competence (boys) +<br>• Social competence (girls) 0<br><br>[a]Game facility was measured through an aggregate measure that included researcher observations of recess behavior, behavior checklists completed by the teacher and researcher, and peer identification of children who were good at sports. |

# Appendix F: Classroom Physical Activity Summary Matrix

Articles describing quasi-experimental or experimental designs are highlighted in the table before the matrix for each setting. Not all studies used these designs.

| Classroom Physical Activity Studies Using Quasi Experimental or Experimental Design (Authors and Date only) | |
|---|---|
| Ahamed, Y., MacDonald, H., Reed, K., Naylor, P.-J., Liu-Ambrose, T., McKay, H. | 2007 |
| Della Valle, J., Dunn, R., Geisert, G., Sinatra, R., Zenhausern, R. | 1986 |
| Fredericks, C.R., Kokot, S.J., Krog, S. | 2006 |
| Maeda, J.K., Randall, L.M. | 2003 |
| Mahar, M.T., Murphy, S.K., Rowe, D.A., Golden, J., Shields, A.T., Raedeke, T.D. | 2006 |
| Molloy, G.N. | 1989 |
| Norlander, T., Moas, L., Archer T. | 2005 |
| Uhrich, T.A., Swalm, R.L. | 2007 |

**Appendix F: Classroom Physical Activity Summary Matrix**[††††]

| Study Citation | Study Focus and Setting | Sample Characteristics | Study Design and Data Collection | Intervention Conditions | Key Outcomes and Results |
|---|---|---|---|---|---|
| Ahamed Y, MacDonald H, Reed K, Naylor P-J, Liu-Ambrose T, McKay H[65]<br><br>School-based physical activity does not compromise children's academic performance.<br><br>*Medicine and Science in Sports and Exercise* 2007;39(2):371-376 | **Study focus:** Classroom<br><br>**Description:** Physical activity intervention evaluation focusing on maintenance and change of academic performance.<br><br>**Setting:** School, physical education<br><br>**Country:** Canada | **Sample 1:** School N: 20<br>**Age range:** NA<br>**Mean age:** NA<br>**Grade:** Primary<br><br>**Sample 2:** Youth N: 288<br>**Age range:** 9–11<br>**Mean age:** 10.2<br>**Grade:** Primary (4th, 5th grades)<br>**Gender:**<br>M: 49.7%<br>F: 50.3%<br>**Ethnicity:**<br>Asian 60.3%<br>White 27.9%<br>Other 11.8% | **Study design:** Experimental<br><br>**Data collection method and time points:** Paper-pencil survey (self-report—moderate to vigorous physical activity as measured by a modified version of the Physical Activity Questionnaire for Children (PAQ-C)<br>⏲ 5 times (baseline minus 3 months, baseline, 3 months, 9 months, 12 months)<br><br>Standardized tests (Canadian Achievement Test-CAT-3 in reading, math and language arts)<br>⏲ 3 times (baseline, 3 months, 12 months) | **Name:** Action Schools! BC (AS! BC) Model<br><br>**Structure:** The AS! BC model complements the 80 minutes per week of physical education time with 15 more minutes per day of physical activity in the classroom (for a total of 75 minutes per week) to achieve the recommended total of 150 minutes per week.<br><br>**Implementation:** The intervention spanned 16 months but academic performance was only evaluated across the school year. Teachers in intervention schools were required to implement classroom-based activities for 15 minutes during each school day. Activities offered by teachers included skipping, dancing, and resistance exercises. | **Did increased physical activity improve academic performance (a combined score of reading, math and language arts)?**<br>• Standardized test score (combined) 0<br><br>**Did increased physical activity improve academic performance by gender?**<br>• Standardized test scores (combined) 0 (by gender) |
| Della Valle J, Dunn R, Geisert G, Sinatra R, Zenhausern R[61]<br><br>The effects of matching and mismatching students' mobility preferences on recognition and memory tasks.<br><br>*Journal of Educational Research* 1986;79(5):267-272 | **Study focus:** Classroom<br><br>**Description:** The effect of activity level on learning<br><br>**Setting:** School, classroom<br><br>**Country:** USA | **Sample 1:** Youth N: 40<br>**Age range:** NR<br>**Mean age:** NR<br>**Grade:** Secondary (junior high school)<br>**Gender:**<br>M: 42.5%<br>F: 57.5%<br>**Ethnicity:** NR | **Study design:** Quasi-experimental<br><br>**Data collection method and time points:** Observation (students studied 15 word pairs in a passive and in an active environment)<br>⏲ 1 time<br><br>Standardized tests (mobility preference—score on element of mobility from learning style assessment)<br>⏲ 1 time<br><br>Standardized tests (word recognition test of 60 word pairs)<br>⏲ 1 time | **Conditions:** Passive condition, active condition<br><br>**Structure:** In the passive condition, students learned word pairs by remaining in their seats while 15 word pairs were flashed on a screen at 4-second intervals. In the active condition, students examined 15 different word pairs printed on cards arranged around the perimeter of the room. Students examined each card for 4 seconds and moved to the next one.<br><br>**Implementation:** Within-subjects design, the same students learned word-pairs in each of the 2 conditions. | **Does matching student's mobility preference to the learning environment improve word recognition?**[i]<br>• Word recognition test score +<br><br>[i]Students who preferred active learning performed significantly better when there was an active learning environment. Students who preferred passive learning performed better in the passive learning environment. When the learning environment matched the student's preferred learning style, scores were significantly better. |

††††Results are coded as follows: + signifies a significant positive outcome; 0 signifies no significant outcome; - signifies a significant negative outcome. Matrices may not include all outcomes described in the article; shaded outcomes are outcomes of primary interest to (and were included in) this review; additional outcomes reported here may be of interest to readers.

NR = Not reported by study authors.

NA = Not applicable.

⏲ Indicates data collection time points.

| Study Citation | Study Focus and Setting | Sample Characteristics | Study Design and Data Collection | Intervention Conditions | Key Outcomes and Results |
|---|---|---|---|---|---|
| Fredericks CR, Kokot SJ, Krog S[66]<br><br>Using a developmental movement programme to enhance academic skills in grade 1 learners.<br><br>*South African Journal for Research in Sport, Physical Education and Recreation* 2006;28(1):29-42 | **Study focus:** Classroom<br><br>**Description:** Movement and academics—interplay between brain and body<br><br>**Setting:** School<br><br>**Country:** South Africa | **Sample 1:** Youth<br>**N:** 53<br>**Age range:** NR<br>**Mean age:** NR<br>**Grade:** Primary (1st grade)<br>**Gender:**<br>M: 43.40%<br>F: 56.60%<br>**Language:**<br>English: 79.3%<br>Africans: 11.3%<br>Other: 9.4% | **Study design:** Experimental<br><br>**Data collection method and time points:** Skill assessment (Aptitude Test for School Beginners—ASB—examined perception, spatial, reasoning, numerical, Gestalt, coordination, memory, and verbal comprehension)<br>⏱ 2 times (baseline, 2 months)<br><br>Standardized test (Draw-a-person—DAP—utilized for emotional indicators)<br>⏱ 2 times (baseline, 2 months) | **Conditions:** Experimental, free-play, educational toys, and control groups.<br><br>**Structure:** The experimental group followed an 8-week movement program with 20 minutes per day. After warm-up, smaller groups were formed to rotate through stations. Activities in stations progressed in difficulty as individual mastery occurred. The freeplay group allowed children to use playground equipment. The educational toys group contained the children in their classrooms, but allowed them to use table-top educational games. The control group followed normal school curriculum.<br><br>**Topics Covered:** Content was of highly specific developmental movements in the developmental sequence of movements through infancy, midline crossing, balance, proprioception, laterality, interhemispheric integration, vestibular work, convergence, divergence, visual accommodation.<br><br>**Training:** Teachers attended a seminar regarding the project and their involvement. | Does exposure to the movement program improve aptitude scores for youth as measured by the Aptitude Test for School Beginners?<br><br>- **Spacial aptitude** +<br>- **Reading aptitude** +<br>- **Math aptitude** +<br>- **Perception** o<br>- **Reasoning** o<br>- **Numerical** o<br>- **Gestalt** o<br>- **Coordination** o<br>- **Memory** o<br>- **Verbal comprehension** o<br>- **Emotional indicators** o |
| Lowden K, Powney J, Davidson J, James C[68]<br><br>*The Class Moves! Pilot in Scotland and Wales: An Evaluation.*<br><br>Edinburgh: Scottish Council for Research in Education; 2001 Jan. Report No.: 100. | **Study focus:** Classroom<br><br>**Description:** Exercises to enhance concentration and motivation<br><br>**Setting:** School, classroom<br><br>**Country:** Scotland and Wales | **Sample 1:** School<br>**N:** 6<br><br>**Sample 2:** Youth<br>**N:** ~192<br>**Age range:** 5–12<br>**Mean age:** NR<br>**Grade:** Primary<br>**Gender:**<br>M: 48%<br>F: 52%<br>**Ethnicity:**<br>**Primarily white** | **Study design:** Case study<br><br>**Data collection method and time points:** Interview (teacher reflection of program impact)<br>⏱ 2 times (baseline, 3 months) | **Name:** The Class Moves! Program<br><br>**Structure:** There were 24 groups of students with a maximum of 8 students in each group. Exercises are grouped by theme and age and are listed on a monthly calendar, which follows a stage-related development plan. Sessions are 10 to 15 minutes and can be conducted before, during, or after any class subject. Ideally activities are a break from sedentary work. | Do teachers report students involved in the Class Moves! Program have increased academic performance measures?[k]<br><br>- Classroom behavior +<br><br>[l]Data collected through qualitative interviews; clear definitions of each outcome were not provided by the authors. |

| Study Citation | Study Focus and Setting | Sample Characteristics | Study Design and Data Collection | Intervention Conditions | Key Outcomes and Results |
|---|---|---|---|---|---|
| | | Sample 3: School personnel N: 24 Sample 4: Parents N: 19 Sample 5: School personnel N: 30 | | | |
| Maeda JK, Randall LM[62] Can academic success come from five minutes of physical activity? *Brock Education Journal* 2003;13(1):14-22 | Study focus: Classroom Description: The impact of adding 5 minutes of physical activity to a day for 2nd-grade students Setting: School, classroom Country: USA | Sample 1: Youth N: 19 Age range: NR Mean age: NR Grade: Primary Gender: M: 36.8% F: 63.2% Ethnicity: NR | Study design: Quasi-experimental, with single subject behavioral design—multiple treatment reversal design Data collection method and time points: Observation (5 minutes running/walking) ⏲ 61 times (each day for 61 days) Teacher-made math fluency test (1-minute math addition test) ⏲ 61 times (each day for 61 days) | Structure: The weekly routine, approximately 1 hour after lunch, 4 days per week, consisted of restroom/water, physical activity, water, and then return to the classroom for the math activity. Implementation: The teacher divided the students into 2 groups based on their performance in math related to addition concepts: 1) grade-level group and 2) below-grade level group. 3 versions of addition problems sheets were used. | Do 5 minutes of a moderate to vigorous activity increase math fluency and concentration (based on teacher observation)? + + • Math fluency • Concentration |
| Mahar MT, Murphy SK, Rowe DA, Golden J, Shields AT, Raedeke TD[63] Effects of a classroom-based program on physical activity and on-task behavior. *Medicine and Science in Sports and Exercise* 2006;38(12): 2086-2094 | Study focus: Classroom Description: A classroom-based physical activity program's effect on elementary school-aged children's physical activity levels and on-task behavior during academic instruction Setting: School, classroom Country: USA | Sample 1: Youth N: 243 Age range: NR Mean age: NR Grade: Primary (K–4th grade) Gender: NR Ethnicity: NR | Study design: Quasi-experimental Data collection method and time points: Structured and timed observation (on-task behavior of 3rd- and 4th-grade students only—defined as verbal or motor behavior that followed class rules and was appropriate to the learning situation) ⏲ Daily over a 12-week period (pre- and postintervention) Measurement device – pedometers (number of steps taken in all K–4th-grade classes) ⏲ 5 days in a week (all children in one grade per week) | Structure: Students in all K–4th-grade classrooms (3 classes per grade) in one school participated in "Energizers." These are classroom-based physical activities that last approximately 10 minutes, integrate grade-appropriate learning materials, involve no equipment, and require little teacher preparation. Training: Before the study, classroom teachers attended a 45-minute training session where they were taught how to lead students through Energizers activities. Training included information about the childhood obesity epidemic. Implementation: Teachers were each asked to lead one 10-minute activity per day for 12 weeks. | Does participation in Energizers increase on-task behavior in school (based on researcher observation)? + • On-task behavior (3rd- and 4th-grade students) Does participation in Energizers increase physical activity in school (based on pedometer counts)? + • Physical activity |

| Study Citation | Study Focus and Setting | Sample Characteristics | Study Design and Data Collection | Intervention Conditions | Key Outcomes and Results |
|---|---|---|---|---|---|
| Molloy GN[64]<br><br>Chemicals, exercise and hyperactivity: a short report.<br><br>*International Journal of Disability, Development and Education* 1989;36(1):57-61 | **Study focus:** Classroom<br><br>**Description:** Effect of exercise on problem solving and attention in normal and hyperactive students<br><br>**Setting:** School, classroom<br><br>**Country:** Australia | **Sample 1:** Youth<br>N: 32<br>**Age range:** NR<br>**Mean age:** NR<br>**Grade:** Primary<br>**Gender:** NR<br>**Ethnicity:** NR | **Study design:** Quasi-experimental<br><br>**Data collection method and time points:** Paper-pencil survey (achievement test scores)<br>⏱ 1 time (immediately following each exercise condition: no exercise, 5 minutes of exercise, 10 minutes of exercise)<br><br>Observation (on-task behavior)<br>⏱ 1 time (immediately following each exercise condition: no exercise, 5 minutes of exercise, 10 minutes of exercise)<br><br>Standardized test (hyperactivity)<br>⏱ 1 time (before study) | **Structure:** Children engaged in 3 levels of aerobic exercise at a constant cadence: no exercise, 5 minutes, or 10 minutes of exercise. | **Does student's participation in 5 minutes of aerobic exercise improve arithmetic problem solving performance?**<br>• Arithmetic performance    +<br>**Does student's participation in 10 minutes of aerobic exercise improve arithmetic problem solving performance?**<br>• Arithmetic performance    0<br>**How does observed attention span change after aerobic exercise?**<br>• Attention    0 |
| Norlander T, Moas L, Archer T[60]<br><br>Noise and stress in primary and secondary school children: noise reduction and increased concentration ability through a short but regular exercise and relaxation program.<br><br>*School Effectiveness and School Improvement* 2005;16(1):91-99 | **Study focus:** Classroom<br><br>**Description:** Relationships between noise, stress, concentration, and exercise<br><br>**Setting:** School, classroom<br><br>**Country:** Sweden | **Sample 1:** Youth<br>N: 84<br>**Age range:** NR<br>**Mean age:** 11.3<br>**Grade:** Cross level (primary and secondary school)<br>**Gender:**<br>M: 45.5%<br>F: 54.5%<br>**Ethnicity:** NR<br><br>**Sample 2:** School personnel<br>N: 7<br>**Mean age:** 42.1<br>**Gender:**<br>M: 28.6%<br>F: 71.4%<br>**Ethnicity:** NR | **Study design:** Quasi-experimental<br><br>**Data collection method and time points:** Measurement device (noise levels in the classroom)<br>⏱ 2 times (baseline, 1 month)<br><br>Paper-pencil survey (student satisfaction with exercise and relaxation program, stress levels)<br>⏱ 2 times (baseline, 1 month)<br><br>Paper-pencil survey (teacher perception of student concentration and stress levels)<br>⏱ 2 times (baseline, 1 month) | **Structure:** Relaxation/exercise episodes occurred twice daily for 4 weeks, immediately following the morning break and after the lunch break. The program took 5 to 10 minutes and consisted of a combination of stretching exercises and relaxation exercises. | **Does the intervention affect student ability to concentrate (as reported by teachers)?**<br>• Concentration    +<br>**Does the intervention reduce classroom noise level (as measured by research staff)?**<br>• Noise levels    +<br>**Does the intervention affect student self-reported stress level?**<br>• Stress level    0 |

| Study Citation | Study Focus and Setting | Sample Characteristics | Study Design and Data Collection | Intervention Conditions | Key Outcomes and Results |
|---|---|---|---|---|---|
| Ulrich TA, Swalm RL[67]<br><br>A pilot study of a possible effect from a motor task on reading performance.<br><br>*Perceptual and Motor Skills* 2007;104(3 Pt 1):1035-1041 | **Study focus:** Classroom<br><br>**Description:** Influence of "cup stacking" and reading achievement<br><br>**Setting:** School, classroom, physical education<br><br>**Country:** USA | **Sample 1:** Youth<br>**N:** 41<br>**Age range:** 10-11<br>**Mean age:** NR<br>**Grade:** Cross level (K-8th grade)<br>**Gender:**<br>**M:** 56%<br>**F:** 44%<br>**Ethnicity:**<br>**Native American:** 1%<br>**Asian-American:** 2%<br>**African-American:** 20%<br>**Latin-American:** 3%<br>**Euro-American:** 74% | **Study design:** Experimental<br><br>**Data collection method and time points:** Standardized tests (measuring reading decoding and comprehension skills using Gates-MacGinitie Reading Test 4th Edition, GMRT-4)<br>🕐 2 times (baseline, 6 weeks)<br><br>Interview (reading instruction fidelity)<br>🕐 1 time (conclusion of intervention) | **Structure:** Five 1-hour lessons modified into 18 20-minute lessons with 3 lessons per week over a period of 6 weeks.<br><br>**Implementation:** Each child had 12 cups to use during the intervention time. Controls had snack time while intervention group "stacked" (intervention group had a later snack time). | Does student participation in sport stacking improve children's reading literacy scores on the GMRT-4 standardized test?<br><br>• **Reading decoding scores**    0<br>• **Reading comprehension**    + |

# Appendix G: Extracurricular Physical Activity Summary Matrix

Articles describing quasi-experimental or experimental designs are highlighted in the table before the matrix for each setting. Not all studies used these designs.

| Extracurricular Physical Activity Studies Using Quasi Experimental or Experimental Design (Authors and Date Only) | |
|---|---|
| Darling, N. | 2005 |
| Reynolds, D., Nicolson, R.I. | 2007 |
| Schumaker, J.F., Small, L., Wood, J. | 1986 |

**Appendix G: Extracurricular Physical Activity Matrix[‡‡‡]**

| Study Citation | Study Focus and Setting | Sample Characteristics | Study Design and Data Collection | Intervention Conditions | Key Outcomes and Results |
|---|---|---|---|---|---|
| Collingwood TR, Sunderlin J, Reynolds R, Kohl HW 3rd[2]<br><br>Physical training as a substance abuse prevention intervention for youth.<br><br>*Journal of Drug Education* 2000; 30(4):435-451 | **Study focus:** Extracurricular physical activity<br><br>**Description:** Fitness as a risk prevention intervention<br><br>**Setting:** School, community<br><br>**Country:** USA | **Sample 1:** Youth<br>N: 34<br>**Mean age:** 15.5<br>**Grade:** Secondary (senior high school)<br>**Gender:**<br>M: 58.8%<br>F: 41.2%<br>**Ethnicity:**<br>Black: 2.9%<br>White: 97.1%<br><br>**Sample 2:** Youth<br>N: 44<br>**Mean age:** 12<br>**Grade:** Secondary (junior high school)<br>**Gender:**<br>M: 53.5%<br>F: 46.5%<br>**Ethnicity:**<br>Black: 15%<br>Hispanic: 3.1%<br>White: 80.4%<br>Other: 1.5% | **Study design:** Descriptive<br><br>**Data collection method and time points:** Fitness test (physical fitness battery)<br>🕒 2 times (baseline, 3 months)<br><br>Paper-pencil survey (self-report of physical activity times per week and rate how compares to peers, self-report of school functioning and grades, self-concept, school attendance, well-being, church participation, relationship with parents, friends' use of cigarettes, alcohol, and drugs)<br>🕒 2 times (baseline, 3 months) | **Name:** First Choice program<br><br>**Training:** Staff were trained as Fitness Leaders in a 40-hour course with a written and practicum certification exam. Content of the staff course focused on fitness assessment techniques, goal setting and exercise prescription, exercise leadership, teaching skills, safety, and foundations content.<br><br>**Structure:** Program was implemented in 22 settings across the state (including 1 juvenile correctional facility, 6 drug treatment facilities, 4 junior high schools, 2 senior high schools, and 9 neighborhood or community centers). This evaluation was conducted in 6 sites (1 high school, 2 junior high schools, and 3 community sites).<br><br>**Method:** There were 24 different modules to teach physical fitness as a life skill, focusing on self-assessment, goal setting, exercise and nutrition planning, and self-reward motivation through exercise classes, educational modules, discussion modules, and individual exercise program maintenance. | **What were the effects of the First Choice fitness program on participating youth academic outcomes and risk factors?**<br><br>Site 1<br>• Grades (self-report)   0<br>• School attendance   0<br>• Self-concept   +<br>Site 2<br>• Grades (self-report)   0<br>• School attendance   0<br>• Self-concept   +<br>Site 3<br>• Grades (self-report)   0<br>• School attendance   0<br>• Self-concept   +<br>Site 4<br>• Grades (self-report)   0<br>• School attendance   0<br>• Self-concept   +<br>Site 5<br>• Grades (self-report)   0<br>• School attendance   0<br>• Self-concept   +<br>Site 6<br>• Grades (self-report)   +<br>• School attendance   +<br>• Self-concept   + |

[‡‡‡]Results are coded as follows: + signifies a significant positive outcome; O signifies no significant outcome; − signifies a significant negative outcome. Matrices may not include all outcomes described in the article; shaded outcomes are outcomes of primary interest to (and were included in) this review; additional outcomes reported here may be of interest to readers.

NR=Not reported by study authors.

🕒 Indicates data collection time points.

| Study Citation | Study Focus and Setting | Sample Characteristics | Study Design and Data Collection | Intervention Conditions | Key Outcomes and Results |
|---|---|---|---|---|---|
| | | **Sample 3:** Youth<br>**N:** 33<br>**Mean age:** 10.9<br>**Grade:** Secondary (junior high school)<br>**Gender:**<br>  **M:** 60%<br>  **F:** 40%<br>**Ethnicity:**<br>  **Hispanic:** 6%<br>  **White:** 94%<br><br>**Sample 4:** Youth<br>**N:** 22<br>**Age range:** NR<br>**Mean age:** 11.4<br>**Grade:** NR (National Guard community site)<br>**Gender:**<br>  **M:** 50%<br>  **F:** 50%<br>**Ethnicity:**<br>  **Black:** 68%<br>  **Hispanic:** 32%<br><br>**Sample 5:** Youth<br>**N:** 40<br>**Mean age:** 11.9<br>**Grade:** NR (National Guard community site)<br>**Gender:**<br>  **M:** 47.5%<br>  **F:** 52.5%<br><br>**Sample 6:** Youth<br>**N:** 156<br>**Mean age:** 11.1<br>**Grade:** NR (National Guard community site)<br>**Gender:**<br>  **M:** 60.8%<br>  **F:** 39.2%<br>**Ethnicity:**<br>  **Black:** 76.2%<br>  **Hispanic:** 3.8%<br>  **White:** 19.8% | | | What were the effects of the First Choice fitness program on participating youth activity levels?[1]<br><br>Site 1<br>• Activity level  0<br>Site 2<br>• Activity level  0<br>Site 3<br>• Activity level  0<br>Site 4<br>• Activity level  0<br>Site 5<br>• Activity level  0<br>Site 6<br>• Activity level  +<br><br>[1]In addition to activity level, other fitness measures included 1-mile run times, sit and reach, sit-ups, push-ups, body fat, and well-being. |

| Study Citation | Study Focus and Setting | Sample Characteristics | Study Design and Data Collection | Intervention Conditions | Key Outcomes and Results |
|---|---|---|---|---|---|
| Crosnoe R[69]<br><br>Academic and health-related trajectories in adolescence: The intersection of gender and athletics.<br><br>*Journal of Health and Social Behavior* 2002; 43(3):317-335 | **Study focus:** Extracurricular physical activity<br><br>**Description:** The relationship of gender and athletics to academic and health-related trajectories in adolescence.<br><br>**Setting:** School<br><br>**Country:** USA | **Sample 1: School**<br>N: 9<br>**Grade:** Secondary (high school)<br><br>**Sample 2:** Youth<br>N: 2,651<br>**Age range:** NR<br>**Mean age:** NR<br>**Grade:** Secondary (high school)<br>**Gender:** NR<br>**Ethnicity:**<br>Ethnic minority: 40%<br>Not specified: 60% | **Study design:** Descriptive, secondary data analysis (see Steinberg et al, 1996)<br><br>**Data collection method and time points:** Paper-pencil survey (self-reported grades, substance use, athletic participation)<br>⏱ 6 times<br>[2 questionnaires answered per year over a 3-year period (1987–1990)]<br><br>Paper-pencil survey (friends' behavior, demographics)<br>⏱ 1 time | No intervention | Do male and female high school student athletes' academic trajectories (based on self-reported grades) improve more than male nonathletes?<br><br>**Start of high school:**<br>• Male athletes + +<br>• Female athletes<br>**Over 3 years:**<br>• Male athletes + +<br>• Female athletes<br><br>Do gender and athlete status affect substance use at the start of high school?<br>• Tobacco, alcohol, or drug use 0<br><br>Are gender and athlete status related to the trajectory of substance use?<br>• Tobacco use 0<br>• Alcohol use (males, female athletes) –<br>• Illegal drug use 0 |
| Darling N, Caldwell LL, Smith R[79]<br><br>Participation in school-based extracurricular activities and adolescent adjustment.<br><br>*Journal of Leisure Research* 2005; 37(1):51-76 | **Study focus:** Extracurricular physical activity<br><br>**Description:** The relationship between school-related extracurricular activities and academic adjustment<br><br>**Setting:** School, after school<br><br>**Country:** USA | **Sample 1:** Youth<br>N: 4,264<br>**Grade:** Secondary (9th–12th grades)<br>**Gender:**<br>M: 47.9%<br>F: 52.1%<br>**Ethnicity:**<br>Asian: 21.3%<br>Black: 4.6%<br>Hispanic: 13.6%<br>White: 60.5%<br><br>**Sample 2 (a subset of sample 1 who participated in longitudinal data collection):** Youth<br>N: 2,462<br>**Grade:** Secondary (9th–12th grades)<br>**Gender:**<br>M: 48%<br>F: 52%<br>**Ethnicity:**<br>Asian: 21.2%<br>Black: 4.4%<br>Hispanic: 13.1%<br>White: 61.3% | **Study design:** Descriptive, secondary analysis of an existing dataset<br><br>**Data collection method and time points:** Paper-pencil survey (participation in extracurricular activity and type of activity, friends' participation in extracurricular activities, attitude towards school, academic aspirations, self-reports on last term grades)<br>⏱ 2 times for Sample 1 (baseline, 12 months)<br>⏱ 1 time for Sample 2 (12 months) | No intervention | Is participation in school-based extracurricular activities (sport and nonsport) associated with indicators of adolescent adjustment (after adjustment for demographics)?[m]<br>• Higher self-reported grades +<br>• Higher academic aspirations +<br>• Positive academic attitudes +<br><br>[m]No significant differences by gender or other demographic characteristics in final analyses. Participants in sports activities had more positive adjustment than nonparticipants in extracurricular activities, but lower positive adjustment than nonsports extracurricular activity participants.<br><br>Do youth who have friends who participate in extracurricular activities have higher indicators of adolescent adjustment?<br>• Higher self-reported grades +<br>• Higher academic aspirations +<br>• Positive academic attitudes + |

| Study Citation | Study Focus and Setting | Sample Characteristics | Study Design and Data Collection | Intervention Conditions | Key Outcomes and Results |
|---|---|---|---|---|---|
| Darling N[78]<br><br>Participation in extracurricular activities and adolescent adjustment: Cross sectional and longitudinal findings.<br><br>*Journal of Youth and Adolescence* 2005; 34(5):493-505 | **Study focus:** Extracurricular physical activity<br><br>**Description:** The relationship between school-related extracurricular activities and academic adjustment<br><br>**Setting:** School, after school<br><br>**Country:** USA | **Sample 1:** School<br>N: 6<br>**Grade:** Secondary (9th–12th grades)<br><br>**Sample 2 (cross-sectional analyses):** Youth<br>N: 3,761<br>**Grade:** Secondary (9th–12th grades)<br>**Gender:**<br>M: 47%<br>F: 53%<br>**Ethnicity:**<br>Asian: 18.7%<br>Black: 4.5%<br>Hispanic: 13.8%<br>White: 64.0%<br><br>**Sample 3 (longitudinal analyses):** Youth<br>N: 3,427<br>**Grade:** Secondary (9th–11th grades) | **Study design:** Quasi-experimental (cross-sectional and longitudinal analyses)<br><br>**Data collection method and time points:** Paper-pencil survey [self-reported grades, attitude towards school, academic aspirations, demographics, engagement in classes, participation in extracurricular activity at school during current year, time spent in extracurricular activities (e.g., interscholastic and intramural sports, performing groups, leadership groups), and clubs, family relationships, parenting behavior, peer relationship, life event stress, depressive symptoms, substance use]<br>⟳ 3 times (1987–1990) | No intervention | Is participation in school-based extracurricular activities associated with indicators of adolescent adjustment (after adjustment for demographics) in year 1 of study?[m]<br><br>• Higher self-reported grades   +<br>• Higher academic aspirations   +<br>• Positive academic attitudes   +<br>• Less depression   0<br><br>"Additional analyses were conducted and in no case did entering time commitment change the association between participation and outcomes. More time spent on extracurricular activities was associated with higher grades and academic aspirations.<br><br>Is participation in school-based extracurricular activities associated with indicators of adolescent adjustment (after adjustment for demographics) across mutiple years of study?[o]<br><br>• Higher self-reported grades   +<br>• Higher academic aspirations   +<br>• Positive academic attitudes   +<br>• Less depression   0<br><br>"Additional analyses were conducted and more years of participation were associated with higher grades, a more positive attitude toward school, and higher academic aspirations.<br><br>Is participation in school-based extracurricular activities associated with indicators of adolescent adjustment (after adjustment for demographics) across mutiple years of study?<br><br>• less drinking   0<br>• less smoking   +<br>• less marijuana use   +<br>• less other drug use   + |

| Study Citation | Study Focus and Setting | Sample Characteristics | Study Design and Data Collection | Intervention Conditions | Key Outcomes and Results |
|---|---|---|---|---|---|
| Fredricks JA, Eccles JS[76]<br><br>Participation in extracurricular activities in middle school years: Are there developmental benefits for African American and European American youth?<br><br>*Journal of Youth and Adolescence* 2008;37:1029-1043 | **Study focus:** Extracurricular physical activity<br><br>**Description:** Extracurricular activities and academic achievement<br><br>**Setting:** Household<br><br>**Country:** USA | **Sample 1:** Youth<br>**N:** 1,047<br>**Age range:** NR<br>**Mean age:** 12.27<br>**Grade:** Secondary (7th, 8th, 11th grades)<br>**Gender:**<br>M: 49%<br>F: 51%<br>**Ethnicity:**<br>Black: 67%<br>White: 33% | **Study design:** Descriptive, secondary analysis of data from the Maryland Adolescent Development in Context Study (MADICS)<br><br>**Data collection method and time points:** Paper-pencil survey and face-to-face interview [self-reported grades, school value, participation in school activities (e.g., clubs, student government, athletic or sports teams at school, and participation in Summer or after-school recreational programs), self-esteem, psychological resiliency, depression, prosocial peers, risky behaviors, race, and gender]<br>🕒 3 times (7th, 8th, and 11th grades) | No intervention | **Did participation in 7th-grade school sports improve academic outcomes at 8th grade?**<br>• Self-reported GPA 0<br>• School value –<br>• Self-esteem 0<br>• Resiliency 0<br>• Depression 0<br><br>**Did participation in 7th-grade school sports improve academic outcomes at 11th grade?**<br>• Self-reported GPA 0<br>• School value –<br>• Self-esteem 0<br>• Resiliency +<br>• Depression 0<br><br>Additional analyses showed a significant effect in 8th grade for race on resiliency and SES on depression; no significant results by gender.<br><br>**Did participation in 7th-grade out-of-school recreation improve academic outcomes at 8th grade?**<br>• Self-reported GPA 0<br>• School value 0<br>• Self-esteem 0<br>• Resiliency +<br>• Depression 0<br><br>**Did participation in 7th-grade out-of-school recreation improve academic outcomes at 11th grade?**<br>• Self-reported GPA 0<br>• School value 0<br>• Self-esteem +<br>• Resiliency 0<br>• Depression 0<br><br>Additional analyses showed no significant effects in 8th or 11th grades for gender, race, or SES.<br><br>**Did participation in 7th-grade school clubs improve academic outcomes at 8th grade?** |

| Study Citation | Study Focus and Setting | Sample Characteristics | Study Design and Data Collection | Intervention Conditions | Key Outcomes and Results |
|---|---|---|---|---|---|
| | | | | | • Self-reported GPA  +<br>• School value  +<br>• Self-esteem  0<br>• Resiliency  +<br>• Depression  0<br><br>Did participation in 7th-grade school clubs improve academic outcomes at 11th grade?<br>• Self-reported GPA  +<br>• School value  0<br>• Self-esteem  0<br>• Resiliency  +<br>• Depression  0<br><br>Additional analyses showed a significant effect in 11th grade for race on GPA and for gender on school value. |
| Fredricks JA, Eccles JS[70]<br><br>Is extracurricular participation associated with beneficial outcomes?: Concurrent and longitudinal relations.<br><br>*Developmental Psychology* 2006; 42(4):698-713 | **Study focus:** Extracurricular physical activity<br><br>**Description:** Extracurricular activities and academic achievement<br><br>**Setting:** Household<br><br>**Country:** USA | **Sample 1:** Youth<br>**N:** 1,075<br>**Age range:** NR<br>**Mean age:** NR<br>**Grade:** Secondary (8th grade—post high school)<br>**Gender:**<br>**M:** 49%<br>**F:** 51%<br>**Ethnicity:**<br>**Black:** 67%<br>**White:** 33% | **Study design:** Descriptive, secondary analysis of data from the Maryland Adolescent Development in Context Study (MADICS)<br><br>**Data collection method and time points:** Combination methods (participation in clubs, sports or prosocial activities)<br>⏱ 3 times (baseline, 3 years, and 5 years—8th grade, 11th grade, and 1 year out of high school)<br><br>Paper-pencil survey (self-reported grades)<br>⏱ 2 times (baseline and 3 years at 8th grade and 11th grade)<br><br>Paper-pencil survey (depression and psychological health, educational expectations, alcohol and drug use, civic engagement)<br>⏱ 3 (baseline, 3 years, and 5 years at 8th grade, 11th grade, and 1 year out of high school) | No intervention | Did participation in high school sports improve academic performance outcomes at 11th grade?<br>• **Self-reported GPA**  +<br>• **Educational expectations**  +<br>• **Self-esteem**  +<br>• **Depression**  +<br>• **Internalizing behavior**  +<br>• **Externalizing behavior**  +<br><br>Did participation in high school sports improve academic performance outcomes 1 year out of high school (controlling for demographics, motivations, and educational expectations)?<br>• School completion  +<br>• Self-esteem  0<br>• Depression  0<br><br>Additional analyses showed no significant results by gender, race, or income for these outcomes. |

| Study Citation | Study Focus and Setting | Sample Characteristics | Study Design and Data Collection | Intervention Conditions | Key Outcomes and Results |
|---|---|---|---|---|---|
| Harrison PA, Narayan G[80]<br><br>Differences in behavior, psychological factors, and environmental factors associated with participation in school sports and other activities in adolescence.<br><br>*Journal of School Health* 2003;73(3):113-120 | **Study focus:** Extracurricular physical activity<br><br>**Description:** Participation in school sports teams, health behavior, psychological factors, environmental factors, and extracurricular activities<br><br>**Setting:** School<br><br>**Country:** USA | **Sample 1:** Youth<br>**N:** 50,168<br>**Age range:** NR<br>**Mean age:** NR<br>**Grade:** Secondary (9th grade)<br>**Gender:**<br>M: 49.3%<br>F: 50.7%<br>**Ethnicity:**<br>American Indian: 1%<br>Asian: 5%<br>Black: 3%<br>Hispanic: 2%<br>White: 82%<br>Unknown: 3%<br>Biracial or multiracial: 4% | **Study design:** Descriptive, secondary analysis of data from the 9th-grade Minnesota Student Survey<br><br>**Data collection method and time points:** Paper-pencil survey [self-report of substance use, antisocial behavior, sexual activity, participation in school sports teams or other activities (e.g., band, choir, volunteer work, clubs or organizations outside of school, etc.), exercise, fruit/vegetable consumption, milk consumption, self-esteem, emotional distress, healthy weight perception, suicidal behavior, family alcohol/problems, victim of physical/sexual abuse, orientation to school, 2-parent family, perceptions of others]<br>⏲ 1 time (2001) | No intervention | Do students who participate in sports only or sports and other activities have significantly higher odds of studying/doing homework and attending class than students who participate in neither sports nor activities?<br>• Doing homework (sports only)[p] +<br>• Doing homework (sports and activities) +<br>• Reduced truancy (sports only) +<br>• Reduced truancy (sports and activities) +<br><br>[p]When the sports-only group was compared to the activities-only group, the activities-only group was significantly more likely to spend time on homework.<br><br>Do students who participate in sports only or sports and other activities have significantly higher odds for school-related psychological and environmental outcomes than students who participate in neither sports nor activities?<br>• Liking school (sports only)[q] +<br>• Liking school (sports and activities) +<br>• Usually feels good about self (sports only) +<br>• Usually feels good about self (sports and activities) +<br>• Believe teachers care a great deal about them (sports only) +<br>• Believe teachers care a great deal about them (sports and activities) +<br><br>[q]When the sports-only group was compared to the activities-only group, the activities-only group was significantly more likely to report liking school.<br><br>Do students who participate in sports only or sports and other activities have significantly higher odds of meeting guidelines for moderate or vigorous exercise than students who participate in neither sports nor activities?<br>• Exercise guidelines (sports only) +<br>• Exercise guidelines (sports and activities) + |

| Study Citation | Study Focus and Setting | Sample Characteristics | Study Design and Data Collection | Intervention Conditions | Key Outcomes and Results |
|---|---|---|---|---|---|
| Hawkins R, Mulkey LM[71]<br><br>Athletic investment and academic resilience in a national sample of African American females and males in the middle grades.<br><br>*Education and Urban Society* 2005;38(1):62-88 | **Study focus:** Extracurricular physical activity<br><br>**Description:** Athletic investment and academic resilience<br><br>**Setting:** School<br><br>**Country:** USA | **Sample 1:** School<br>**N:** 1,052<br>**Grade:** Secondary (8th grade)<br><br>**Sample 2:** Youth<br>**N:** 2,217<br>**Age range:** 13–16<br>**Mean age:** NR<br>**Grade:** Secondary (8th grade)<br>**Gender:**<br>**M:** 49.8%<br>**F:** 50.2%<br>**Ethnicity:** NR | **Study design:** Descriptive, secondary analysis of base year data from the National Educational Longitudinal Study of 1988 (NELS88)<br><br>**Data collection method and time points:** Paper-pencil survey (student self-reported level of participation in interscholastic and intramural sports; plans to enroll in high school academic or college preparatory track, graduate high school, or attend college; report of how popular or important they are viewed to be among schoolmates, student report of behavior or academic referrals, self-reported absenteeism, tardiness, class preparedness, school anticipation)<br>⏱ 1 time (February to June, 1988)<br><br>Paper-pencil survey (teacher ratings of student performance/ability)<br>⏱ 1 time (February to June, 1988) | No intervention | **Does participating in interscholastic sports improve educational plans, peer status, and academic investments?**<br><br>• Academic ability (teacher rating of males)  0<br>• Academic ability (teacher rating of females)  0<br>• Enroll in academic track (males)  +<br>• Enroll in academic track (females)  0<br>• Graduate from high school (males)  +<br>• Graduate from high school (females)  +<br>• Attend college (males)  0<br>• Attend college (females)  0<br>• Social misconduct (males)  0<br>• Social misconduct (females)  0<br>• Attendance problems (males)  0<br>• Attendance problems (females)  0<br>• Academic unpreparedness (males)  0<br>• Academic unpreparedness (females)  0<br>• Interest in classes (males)  +<br>• Interest in classes (females)  +<br><br>**Does participating in intramural sports improve educational plans, peer status, and academic investments?**<br><br>• Academic ability (teacher rating of males)  +<br>• Academic ability (teacher rating of females)  0<br>• Enroll in academic track (males)  +<br>• Enroll in academic track (females)  0<br>• Graduate from high school (males)  +<br>• Graduate from high school (females)  0<br>• Attend college (males)  +<br>• Attend college (females)  0<br>• Social misconduct (males)  0<br>• Social misconduct (females)  0<br>• Attendance problems (males)  0<br>• Attendance problems (females)  0<br>• Academic unpreparedness (males)  0<br>• Academic unpreparedness (females)  0<br>• Interest in classes (males)  +<br>• Interest in classes (females)  0 |

| Study Citation | Study Focus and Setting | Sample Characteristics | Study Design and Data Collection | Intervention Conditions | Key Outcomes and Results |
|---|---|---|---|---|---|
| McNeal, RB[77]<br><br>Extracurricular activities and high school dropouts<br><br>*Sociology of Education* 1995; 68(1):62-81 | **Study focus:** Extracurricular physical activity<br><br>**Description:** Extracurricular activities and school dropout rates<br><br>**Setting:** School<br><br>**Country:** USA | **Sample 1:** Schools<br>**N:** 735<br>**Grade:** Secondary (9th–12th grades)<br><br>**Sample 2:** Youth<br>**N:** 14,249<br>**Age range:** NR<br>**Mean age:** 15.5<br>**Grade:** Secondary (9th–12th grade)<br>**Gender:**<br>M: 48%<br>F: 52%<br>**Ethnicity:**<br>Black: 9.4%<br>Hispanic: 9.5%<br>Other: 2.2%<br>White: 78.9% | **Study design:** Descriptive, secondary analysis of data from the High School and Beyond (HSB) dataset<br><br>**Data collection method and time points:** Paper-pencil survey and face-to-face interview (self-reported grades; school value; participation in school activities such as clubs, student government, athletic or sports teams at school, and Summer or after-school recreational programs; self-esteem; psychological resiliency; depression; prosocial peers; risky behaviors; race; and gender)<br><br>⏱ 2 times (baseline in 1980 and 2 year follow-up in 1982) | No intervention | **Does participation in athletics decrease high school dropout rates?**<br>• **Lower dropout rates**    +<br><br>Additional subgroup analyses were conducted without significance testing; it appears that participation may further decrease dropout probability for blacks, and higher SES students. Additional analyses showed that when students participate in more than one activity, little is gained; athletic participation is the only one that remains significant.<br><br>**Did participation in other nonsports extracurricular activities decrease dropout rates?**<br>• Fine arts    ○<br>• Academic clubs    ○<br>• Vocational clubs    ○<br><br>Analyses also controlled for how much time students spent working during the school year. |
| Reynolds D, Nicolson RI[34]<br><br>Follow-up of an exercise-based treatment for children with reading difficulties.<br><br>*Dyslexia* 2007;13(2):78-96 | **Study focus:** Extracurricular physical activity<br><br>**Description:** Exercise-based treatment for children with reading difficulties<br><br>**Setting:** Household<br><br>**Country:** United Kingdom | **Sample 1:** School<br>**N:** 1<br>**Grade:** Primary<br><br>**Sample 2:** Youth<br>**N:** 35<br>**Age range:** NR<br>**Mean age:** 9<br>**Grade:** Primary (UK junior school)<br>**Gender:**<br>M: 54.3%<br>F: 45.7%<br>**Ethnicity:** NR | **Study design:** Quasi-experimental<br><br>**Data collection method and time points:** Standardized tests (cognitive and motor skills—dyslexia screening test)<br><br>⏱ 4 times (June 2000, June 2001, June 2002, and June 2003)<br><br>Standardized tests (school-administered tests)<br><br>⏱ 3 times (June 2001, June 2002, and June 2003) | **Structure:** Participants were assigned to the intervention or comparison group matched on the basis of age, and dyslexia 'at-risk' levels.<br><br>**Structure:** Intervention: youth participated in the DDAT (dyslexia, dyspraxia and attention-deficit disorder treatment) exercise-based daily treatment at home for 6 months. Comparison: youth had no additional activity. | **Did exposure to the exercise program improve youth's performance in motor and verbal skills over time?**<br>• **Rapid naming**    +<br>• **Bead threading**    +<br>• **1-minute reading**    ○<br>• **Postural stability**    +<br>• **Phonemic segmentation**    +<br>• **2-minute spelling**    ○<br>• **Backwards digit span**    +<br>• **Nonsense passage reading**    ○<br>• **1-minute writing**    ○<br>• **Verbal fluency**    ○<br>• **Semantic fluency**    +<br><br>The intervention group made roughly normal progress per year posttreatment compared with the projected mean pretreatment. |

| Study Citation | Study Focus and Setting | Sample Characteristics | Study Design and Data Collection | Intervention Conditions | Key Outcomes and Results |
|---|---|---|---|---|---|
| Schumaker JF, Small L, Wood J[72]<br><br>Self-concept, academic achievement, and athletic participation.<br><br>*Perceptual and Motor Skills* 1986; 62(2):387-390 | **Study focus:** Extracurricular physical activity<br><br>**Description:** Effects of athletic participation on self-concept and academic achievement in high school subjects<br><br>**Setting:** After school<br><br>**Country:** USA | **Sample 1:** Youth<br>**N:** 85<br>**Age range:** NR<br>**Mean age:** NR<br>**Grade:** Secondary (12th grade)<br>**Gender:**<br>M: 50.6%<br>F: 49.4%<br>**Ethnicity:** NR | **Study design:** Quasi-experimental<br><br>**Data collection method and time points:** Administrative records (grades)<br>🕐 1 time<br><br>Paper-pencil survey (self-concept questionnaire, participation for at least 2 years in a varsity sport)<br>🕐 1 time | No intervention | Does athletic participation improve school-reported grades and student-reported self-concept?<br><br>• **Grades**   0<br>• **Self-concept**   +<br><br>Does athletic participation improve school-reported grades and student-reported self-concept?<br><br>• Grades (males)   0<br>• Grades (females)   0<br>• Self-concept (males)   +<br>• Self-concept (females)   0 |
| Spence JC, Poon P[73]<br><br>Results from the Alberta Schools' Athletic Association Survey.<br><br>*Research Update* (serial online) 1997, September; 5(1) | **Study focus:** Extracurricular physical activity<br><br>**Description:** Survey results on sports participation in Alberta schools<br><br>**Setting:** School<br><br>**Country:** Alberta, Canada | **Sample 1:** School<br>**N:** 36<br>**Grade:** Secondary (high school)<br><br>**Sample 2:** Youth<br>**N:** 883<br>**Age range:** NR<br>**Mean age:** 18<br>**Grade:** Secondary (high school)<br>**Gender:**<br>M: 50.3%<br>F: 49.7%<br>**Ethnicity:** NR | **Study design:** Descriptive<br><br>**Data collection method and time points:** Paper-pencil survey (self-report of school grades, school-based sports participation, nonschool sports participation, extracurricular activity, substance use, and criminal offenses)<br>🕐 1 time | No intervention | Does participation in school-based sports improve students' self-reported academic achievement?<br><br>• **Self-reported grades**   + |
| Stephens LJ, Schaben LA[74]<br><br>The effect of interscholastic sports participation on academic achievement of middle level school students.<br><br>*NASSP Bulletin* 2002; 86(630):34-41 | **Study focus:** Extracurricular physical activity<br><br>**Description:** The relationship between academic achievement and participation in interscholastic sports<br><br>**Setting:** School, classroom<br><br>**Country:** USA | **Sample 1:** Youth<br>**N:** 136<br>**Age range:** NR<br>**Mean age:** NR<br>**Grade:** Secondary (8th grade)<br>**Gender:**<br>M: 50%<br>F: 50%<br>**Ethnicity:** NR | **Study design:** Descriptive<br><br>**Data collection method and time points:** Standardized tests (math portion of the California Achievement Test—CAT)<br>🕐 1 time<br><br>Paper-pencil survey (interscholastic sports participation)<br>🕐 1 time<br><br>Administrative records (math grade and cumulative grades)<br>🕐 1 time | No intervention | Do athletes have better academic outcomes than nonathletes?<br><br>• **Math grades**   +<br>• **Math CAT scores**   +<br>• **Overall GPA**   +<br><br>• GPA (male athletes compared with male nonathletes)   +<br>• GPA (female athletes compared with female nonathletes)   +<br>• GPA (female athletes compared with male athletes)   + |

| Study Citation | Study Focus and Setting | Sample Characteristics | Study Design and Data Collection | Intervention Conditions | Key Outcomes and Results |
|---|---|---|---|---|---|
| Yin Z, Moore JB[75]<br><br>Re-examining the role of interscholastic sport participation in education.<br><br>*Psychological Reports* 2004; 94(3 Pt 2):1447-1454 | **Study focus:** Extracurricular physical activity<br><br>**Description:** Relationship between interscholastic sports and dropout rate, cognitive score, locus of control, and self-concept<br><br>**Setting:** School, schoolwide<br><br>**Country:** USA | **Sample 1:** Youth<br>**N:** 1,883<br>**Age range:** NR<br>**Mean age:** NR<br>**Grade:** Cross level (8th–12th grades)<br>**Gender:** NR<br>**Ethnicity:** NR | **Study design:** Descriptive, secondary analysis of data from the base year and follow-ups 1 and 2 of the National Educational Longitudinal Study of 1988 (NELS88)<br><br>**Data collection method and time points:** Standardized tests (composite score of math and reading standardized tests)<br>⏲ 3 times (baseline, 24 months, 48 months)<br><br>Paper-pencil survey—NELS (interscholastic sport participation, self-concept, locus of control)<br>⏲ 3 times (baseline, 24 months, 48 months)<br><br>Administrative records (school records of dropouts)<br>⏲ 1 time (48 months–12th grade) | No intervention | Does interscholastic sport participation impact student self-report of locus of control and self-concept?<br><br>• 8th-grade locus of control + <br>• 10th-grade locus of control + <br>• 12th-grade locus of control 0 <br>• 8th-grade self-concept + <br>• 10th-grade self-concept + <br>• 12th-grade self-concept 0 <br><br>Does interscholastic sport participation improve a composite score of reading and math standardized test scores?<br><br>• 8th-grade composite test score − <br>• 10th-grade composite test score 0 <br>• 12th-grade composite test score 0 <br><br>Does participation in interscholastic sport in 8th grade decrease student dropout rates reported by school administration?<br><br>• Dropout rate (boys) + <br>• Dropout rate (girls) + <br><br>Does participation in interscholastic sport in 10th grade decrease student dropout rates reported by school administration?<br><br>• Dropout rate (boys) + <br>• Dropout rate (girls) + |